ObamaCare
Survival Guide

ObamaCare
Survival Guide

NICK J. TATE

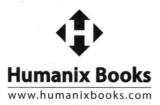

Humanix Books
www.humanixbooks.com

Humanix Books
ObamaCare Survival Guide

© 2013 by Nick J. Tate
A Humanix Books publication
First Edition

Humanix Books
P.O. Box 20989
West Palm Beach, FL 33416
USA
www.humanixbooks.com
email: info@humanixbooks.com

Humanix Books is a division of Humanix Publishing LLC. Its trademark, consisting of the words "Humanix Books" is registered in the U.S. Patent and Trademark Office and in other countries.

Printed in the United States of America and the United Kingdom.

Library of Congress Cataloging-in-Publication Data

Tate, Nicholas, 1959-
Obamacare survival guide : the patient protection and affordable care act and how it affects you and your healthcare / Nicholas Tate.—First edition.
    pages cm
Includes index.
ISBN 978-0-89334-862-5 (pbk.) — ISBN 978-0-89334-909-7 (e-book)
1. Health care reform–United States. 2. Medical policy–United States. 3. Medical care–United States. 4. Medical care, Cost of–United States–Forecasting. I. Title.
RA395.D44T38 2012
362.10973—dc23
2012034031

This book is dedicated to the American people.

TABLE OF CONTENTS

ToC

Chapter 3:
ObamaCare: A Multiyear Timetable   **29**

Added December 2012

PREFACE

T HE PATIENT PROTECTION AND AFFORDABLE CARE ACT, signed into law by President Barack Obama, has been called the most important piece of health-related legislation in U.S. history. And yet today, most Americans still have many practical questions about how it is likely to affect their lives, pocketbooks, and healthcare:

- Will ACA's provisions raise insurance costs and premiums?

- How is it going to change the way doctors, hospitals, and insurers do business?

- Are the law's requirements likely to improve the nation's health as a whole?

- How will it affect uninsured Americans? Employers? Working families? Those on Medicare or Medicaid? Young people? Seniors and nursing home residents?

In essence, this book was written to answer these questions, and provide some context on the law's passage, to show which early ACA provisions are already in play, what lies ahead and how the nation's healthcare system will be fundamentally transformed by what has come to be known as ObamaCare over the next decade.

Regardless of your political views on the new law — whether you like what it aims to do, whether you believe it is a step in the right direction or the wrong way for the nation to go — this book goes beyond the sound bites and headlines to provide a detailed analysis of what it will mean for you and other American healthcare consumers.

What we've tried to present is a concise guide to the nearly 500 provisions contained in the ACA legislation. And while some aspects of the law may be altered by future election results, congressional action and the decisions of federal and state officials charged with implementing ACA's requirements, one thing is clear: Significant healthcare changes have already been set in motion and will continue in the years ahead — shifts that will touch virtually every American.

This book aims to provide a guide to those changes, with a specific focus on consumer impacts.

Part I details how ObamaCare stacks up to other major social legislation, including Social Security and Medicare, with a timetable of key events in ACA's development, and an outline of what the law means for specific groups of Americans.

Part II provides an overview of the law's goals to reduce the ranks of the nation's uninsured, including sections on the individual mandate, expansion of Medicaid, new health insurance exchanges that will be set up for individual policyholders, and financial incentives for small businesses to provide coverage for workers.

Part III examines new consumer protections in ObamaCare, the impact on Medicare recipients, and several pilot programs that aim to test new healthcare approaches designed to improve quality and cut costs at the same time.

Part IV takes a closer look at ACA's provisions for boosting Americans' overall health and pushing preventive care programs, as well as unresolved questions about long-term care and what's likely to be included in the prescribed list of "essential health benefits" all insurers will be required to provide.

Part V digs into ObamaCare's costs, following the money to detail how ACA's provisions will largely be funded, who will be most affected, and the possible ripple effects on other programs.

Part VI offers a practical guide to how to make good decisions in the changing healthcare marketplace — whether you are self-employed, receiving public assistance, working for a large or small company, using prescription medicines, or have a pre-existing condition.

Sprinkled throughout the book are key facts and figures, quotes and good advice — all designed to help deepen your understanding of ACA. On the pages that follow you will learn:

- Why the U.S. Supreme Court's ruling to uphold ObamaCare wasn't a complete victory for the White House and could complicate the way key aspects of ACA are implemented by the states.

- How health insurance costs have already changed for many American families since the law's passage.

- Why tens of millions of Americans continue to have no health insurance and what the new law proposes to address that reality.

- What new rights and advantages you will have under the law if you have a pre-existing health condition, are self-employed, run your own company, or your insurer suddenly drops your coverage.

- The good news and bad news ObamaCare poses for those who currently have health insurance — from the host of new consumer protections to what you will have to pay for your coverage.

- How various segments of the healthcare industry — doctors, nurses, clinicians, hospital administrators, nursing home operators, drug companies and insurers — will be affected by the law.

- What ObamaCare means for the roughly 150 million Americans who receive their health insurance through their employer.

- How new state-based health insurance exchanges, slated to open in 2014, will offer subsidized insurance coverage to individuals who fail to qualify for Medicaid or Medicare or are not covered through employer-based plans.

- What it may mean if you don't obtain health insurance when the individual mandate takes effect.

- Your options if you're a young adult — under the age of 30 — and don't have health coverage.

- What ObamaCare opponents in states such as Florida and Texas are doing to thwart the requirements of the new law, and how that could affect residents of those and other states.

- How the new law deals with controversial insurance issues — including coverage for contraception and abortions.

- What "essential health benefits" insurance companies will be required to provide.

- How new programs have already been created to help adults with pre-existing conditions who are in desperate need of health insurance, and what you can do to take advantage of them.

■ How to determine if new "means testing" provisions, expanded under Medicare, might affect your pocketbook if you are a senior.

■ What the new laws do — and don't do — to curb rising medical costs in the United States.

In short, this book has been produced as a thinking person's guide to ObamaCare — chock-full of insightful analysis, clear-eyed perspectives and practical consumer advice.

Whether you're a senior, college student, small business owner, corporate executive, unemployed, uninsured or have a pre-existing condition, these pages can help you make smarter decisions about your healthcare — and your healthcare dollar.

As a more informed healthcare consumer, you'll be empowered to improve the quality of your life — and perhaps even extend it.

For More Information

To get the latest updates on the ObamaCare law and its impact on you, sign up for free email alerts by going to *www.SurvivingObamaCare.com.*

PART I

ObamaCare: The Essentials

> **"**It's not an exaggeration to say that if the new healthcare system becomes fully operational in a few years it will change the way all of us live.**"**

WELCOME TO OBAMACARE 1

On March 23, 2010, President Barack Obama signed into law a sweeping reform of the nation's healthcare system, handing down to the American people with a stroke of his pen the Patient Protection and Affordable Care Act — one of the most significant and controversial pieces of social legislation in the history of the United States (we will refer to it simply as "ObamaCare" throughout this book, a label that is hardly a pejorative since President Obama himself has endorsed its use).

ObamaCare's Rough Rollout

It's not an exaggeration to say that if the new healthcare system becomes fully operational in a few years it will change the way all of us live. That's because it fundamentally restructures the delivery of healthcare in our nation — a system everyone must rely on to some degree during the course of his or her life.

Numerous political challenges, beyond the 2012 November election results, could delay or halt implementation of key provisions of the law.

Predictions about ObamaCare's demise have abounded since it came into being, but thus far the controversial law has proven itself remarkably durable, not only in surviving a brutal legislative battle to win congressional approval, but also in overcoming numerous obstacles and setbacks since then, the biggest of which was the legal challenge mounted by 26 state governments.

It took two years for the lawsuit brought by these states to work its way through the federal court system, but the controversial case was finally resolved in June 2012 when the Supreme Court of the United States handed down its decisive ruling. It decided in favor of the Obama administration on nearly all the legal points of contention and, most important of all, upheld the so-called "individual mandate" provision of the law, which compels every American to obtain health insurance or pay a fine.

> **? DID YOU KNOW . . .**
>
> **The Supreme Court's ruling wasn't all good news for the White House. It ruled by a 7-2 vote that the federal government could not, in the words of Chief Justice John Roberts, put "a gun to the head" of individual states to force them to expand Medicaid coverage within their borders against their will.**

The Supreme Court ruled by a narrow 5-4 majority that the individual mandate was constitutional under the federal government's power to impose taxes on citizens. This was a gigantic victory for the law's supporters because the individual mandate is ObamaCare's central pillar — an essential structural support that holds the new healthcare system together. Had it been struck down by the court, it is probable that the entire law would have fallen with it.

The Supreme Court's ruling, however, wasn't all good news for the White House. It also ruled by a 7-2 vote that the federal government could not, in the words of Chief Justice John Roberts, put "a gun to the head" of individual states to force them to expand Medicaid coverage within their borders against their will. ObamaCare had stipulated that individual states must let more of their citizens into the program or risk losing the federal matching funds that pay for more than half of Medicaid's cost in each state.

The first part of the court's ruling gives ObamaCare a constitutional stamp of approval, permitting it to move forward in all its complexity; the second part weakens its power significantly by taking away the big financial stick designed to coerce states to expand their Medicaid programs. The court, however, leaves untouched the generous financial carrot that the law also includes to achieve the same end.

The federal government currently pays on average 57 percent of the cost of current Medicaid enrollees in each state. Realizing that maintaining this level of financial support would not be enough of an incentive for states to expand Medicaid within their borders to cover more people, the authors of ObamaCare decided to pay much more of the cost for those "newly eligible" for the program than it now pays for current enrollees.

According to the Congressional Budget Office, each state will have about 93 percent of the cost of these "new eligibles" covered by the federal government from 2014 to 2020 — a large increase over the current 57 percent federal funding level for Medicaid.

This appears to be a sweet deal for the states to significantly increase the number of insured within their borders and have the federal government pay for nearly all of their health coverage. Some Republican governors, including Rick Perry of Texas and Rick Scott of Florida, however, have raised legitimate concerns. They wonder what will happen to the federal contribution after 2020. Given the budgetary mess in Washington, they worry that the financial burden could be shifted back onto state governments at that time, or even sooner, if Congress suddenly decides to change the current law.

Governors like Perry and Scott are also concerned about a flood of new Medicaid enrollees who sign up because the individual mandate forces them to, but who fall under the old eligibility requirements. This so-called "woodwork effect" could amount to a very large expense for states because the federal government will pay for these "old eligibles" under the old formula, meaning that states will get only 57 percent of their cost covered by Washington rather than the 93 percent level for the "new eligibles."

Perry's and Scott's fears are justified in light of a scholarly analysis of the "woodwork effect" published in 2010 in the *New England Journal of Medicine* by Ben Sommers and Arnold Epstein. According to their estimate, only 62 percent of the people who are eligible for Medicaid nationwide right now have actually signed up for the program — fewer than two out of every three. Participation rates are much lower in Texas (48 percent) and Florida (44 percent), meaning the financial impact from the sudden enrollment of large numbers of "old eligibles" will be even greater in those states.

With state budgets already strained to the breaking point everywhere in the country and Medicaid typically accounting for one in four dollars a state spends, the potential impact of ObamaCare on state balance sheets cannot be overstated, even with the generous financial support pledged by the federal government to help expand Medicaid through 2020.

> **" I think Wall Street looks at [the states resisting ObamaCare's Medicaid expansion] and says, 'Wait a minute, these guys are nuts.' The market has been looking at the Republican governors' statements as just political."**
> — Richard Evans,
>   Analyst at Sector
>   & Sovereign Research

Having said this, in the end, most states will probably fall in line and agree to accept ObamaCare's expansion of Medicaid. The gigantic amount of federal dollars that are now within their reach will be difficult to resist over the long term. As Richard Evans, an analyst at Sector & Sovereign Research, put it: "I think Wall Street looks at [the states resisting ObamaCare's Medicaid expansion] and says, 'Wait a minute, these guys are nuts.' The market has been looking at the Republican governors' statements as just political."

Viewed from a historical perspective, there is good reason to believe that resistant states will eventually get on board with the program's expansion. When Medicaid was signed into law in 1965 only six states agreed to participate, but by 1982 every state had joined (Arizona was the last holdout). It took

17 years to get full participation in the program, but eventually that goal was reached — an outcome likely to be repeated if ObamaCare survives over the long haul.

ObamaCare's Durability

With the individual mandate upheld as constitutional by the Supreme Court, ObamaCare has been given a green light. The law is moving forward, albeit slowed somewhat by the new power given to the states to opt out of the expansion of Medicaid if they choose. But this is a road bump rather than a stop sign and in the long run will not prevent the new healthcare system from becoming fully operational.

> **? DID YOU KNOW . . .**
> ObamaCare's support in the House (219-212) and Senate (56-44) was tenuous at best, especially since it became law without a single vote from the opposition party.

All told ObamaCare has, like the proverbial cat with nine lives, survived multiple death scares. When it was being debated in Congress, it seemed many times to hang by a gossamer thread, and yet ultimately won approval in the U.S. Senate after an extraordinary procedural maneuver to block a Republican filibuster that would have certainly killed it in the legislative cradle.

ObamaCare made it out of Congress and onto the desk of President Obama, but just barely. It became the law of the land when he signed it, but since then has not gained any appreciable momentum beyond surviving repeated legal and political assaults. It has remained unpopular with the American people, a majority of whom have consistently said they wish it were repealed.

According to the respected pollster, Rasmussen Reports, ObamaCare remains as unpopular today as when it became law — a level that has remained unchanged even after the Supreme Court's decision gave it an injection of legitimacy from the third branch of government (see Table 1-1).

TAB. 1-1: **PERCENTAGE FAVORING REPEAL OF OBAMACARE**	
	% Of American People Favoring Repeal of ObamaCare*
July 2012 (After Supreme Court ruling)	52%
January 2012	52%
July 2011	57%
January 2011	53%
July 2010	52%
March 2010 (ObamaCare becomes law)	55%

Source: Rasmussen Reports. Each data point is based on a representative sample of the U.S. population, with a sample size of 1,000. The margin of error is +/- 3 points.

Right from the beginning, ObamaCare has defied the odds. Its passage without the public behind it was unusual in itself, but even more so when measured against historical precedents for similar social legislation like Social Security and Medicare, both of which enjoyed widespread popular support and garnered strong bipartisan votes in Congress.

Social Security, for instance, was voted into law by huge majorities in both the House of Representatives (372-33 in favor) and the Senate (77-6). Medicare also won bipartisan majorities, with vote tallies of 313-115 in the House and 68-21 in the Senate. Against these historic bipartisan benchmarks, ObamaCare's support in the House (219-212) and Senate (56-44) was tenuous at best, especially since it became law without a single vote from the opposition party.

Even though ObamaCare was passed in a heavy-handed fashion that is unprecedented, its enduring unpopularity has surprised some informed observers. During the national debate over the law prior to its passage, former President Bill Clinton predicted that "the minute the president signs the healthcare reform bill, approval will go up because Americans are inherently optimistic." Clinton later admitted he was wrong.

Weak at its birth, ObamaCare nonetheless survived its next biggest test by another razor-thin vote when it was upheld by the Supreme

Court. Had Chief Justice John Roberts voted the other way, the individual mandate would have been struck down, and probably the entire law with it.

Despite the Supreme Court's upholding of the law, the rollout of several early provisions of ObamaCare has not been without controversy. In case you missed them, here are some of the big developments since the law's passage in early 2010:

- **Contraception Mandate** — The decision of the Obama administration to mandate contraception coverage for women, enabling them to obtain it without a co-pay under their insurance plans, created a whirlwind of anger from religious organizations who have moral qualms about the issue. Roman Catholics, in particular, objected to the mandate as an infringement of their religious liberty as guaranteed by the Constitution. Although the White House has backed off its initial rule, granting some waivers and allowing religious organizations to shift the contraception coverage decision into the hands of insurers, the controversy continues in the court system. As of late summer, 23 lawsuits had been filed against the contraception mandate, but a final judicial ruling about the issue was still a long way off.

- **No More CLASS** — Also known as "Community Living Assistance and Supports," this highly controversial part of ObamaCare was officially suspended by the White House in October 2011. A well-intentioned insurance plan designed to provide financial help for the long-term care of those who need assistance with basic living tasks made difficult with age

> **? DID YOU KNOW . . .**
> According to a study by the independent Kaiser Family Foundation, health insurance premiums rose 9% for families in 2011 to a level that now exceeds $15,000 on average per year — the biggest annual spike upward since 2004.

or disability, CLASS needed to prove that it could pay for itself entirely through enrollee contributions before it could begin operating. Unable to dispel fears that enrollment levels would be very low (participation was voluntary) and that taxpayers would end up funding yet another budget-busting entitlement, the administration was forced to put CLASS in mothballs, where it remains today, not officially repealed but effectively dead.

- **Rising Healthcare Costs** — One of the biggest goals of ObamaCare was to decrease (or at least control) healthcare costs, which have been rising rapidly in recent years. On this metric the new law has thus far completely failed as costs are now actually rising at a faster rate than seen before it passed. According to a study by the independent Kaiser Family Foundation, health insurance premiums rose 9 percent for families in 2011 to a level that now exceeds $15,000 on average per year — the biggest annual spike upward since 2004. Deductibles have also significantly increased as employers have shifted a greater financial burden for health insurance onto the shoulders of their workers. President Obama has obviously fallen far short of his 2008 campaign promise in which he assured Americans that his healthcare plan "would save the average family $2,500 on their premiums."

- **Non-Compliance Waivers** — After the heavy weight of new ObamaCare mandates fell on the backs of businesses, many were pushed by the skyrocketing insurance costs to the brink of dropping healthcare coverage for their workers. Rather than see the number of uninsured Americans suddenly increase by millions as a result, the White House has as of mid-2012 granted 1,625 non-compliance waivers affecting almost four million people, permitting hard-pressed companies and labor unions that have obtained them to sidestep the costly mandates for a limited time. The administration has asserted that waivers will no longer be necessary once the biggest parts of ObamaCare take effect in 2014, but that remains to be seen. The hope is that the expansion of health insurance coverage to millions of more people at that time will create economies of scale, put downward pressure on costs and make the ObamaCare mandates easier for businesses to swallow.

Deciphering ObamaCare

As healthcare consumers, all Americans are interested in understanding the impact ObamaCare will have on their own lives and the lives of their families. But if you're bewildered by ObamaCare's tangled complexities and murky provisions, you're not alone. According to a survey conducted by the Kaiser Family Foundation, 53 percent of Americans said they were "confused" by the new healthcare system. And among the 47 percent who claim to understand it well enough, their depth of knowledge about the law will in many cases be shallower than they believe.

Americans simply are not paying close attention to ObamaCare as shown by a Pew Research Center survey conducted after the landmark Supreme Court ruling on the law. When asked what they thought of the ruling, 30 percent of the people surveyed admitted their ignorance of what the court had decided and another 15 percent said they thought the court had overturned the law when, in fact, it had done precisely the opposite. Combine these numbers, and about one out of every two citizens admits to not paying attention to the law.

For most of us, ObamaCare remains just as much of a mystery today as when it was being created behind the closed doors of the White House and Congress. But now that the Supreme Court has upheld the law, the time has come for us to take a closer look at ObamaCare, and what it really

! GOOD ADVICE:

If you know little about healthcare beyond what you and your family have personally dealt with in the current system and want to learn about ObamaCare, this book is for you. It gives a broad overview of the new law and describes its most important parts.

means for us as individuals and for our nation as a whole.

This book was written to help you with that discovery process. It's for regular people who want to know more about ObamaCare, but don't have the time or the inclination to sort through the overwhelming mishmash of details that makes it so difficult to comprehend.

If you know little about healthcare beyond what you and your family have personally dealt with in the current system and want to learn about ObamaCare, this book is for you. It gives a broad overview of the new law and describes its most important parts (healthcare isn't the most exciting topic in the world, but given its importance in our lives it certainly demands our attention).

Unfortunately, we can't give you every detail about ObamaCare. That's because the official document that contains the new law is as impenetrably dense as a large county's White Pages. At a daunting 2,500 pages or so, it contains endless paragraphs of mind-numbing legalese that only an army of meticulous lawyers would be able to decipher — most of it with no relevance to you.

If that weren't enough arcane minutiae to digest, the finer points of the law have yet to be written. You read that correctly. Executive branch agencies like the U.S. Department of Health and Human Services have yet to create many of the rules and regulations needed to make the new healthcare system run. The White House's new contraception mandate announced in early 2012 is an example of how important and controversial these decisions can be.

ObamaCare is thus very much a work in progress — a newborn law that will continue to grow and mutate before it matures into a fully-fledged presence in our lives, assuming it is not repealed or blunted by a future president and Congress. Whether it is able to survive or not, the passionate national discussion about how to fix the problems that beset healthcare in the United States is not likely to end any time soon, making this book a valuable resource, regardless of ObamaCare's fate.

If ObamaCare passes electoral tests and congressional scrutiny in the years to come, its critics will remain marginalized but still loud enough to be heard. If ObamaCare, on the other hand, is drained of its force, the problems that it sought to fix will also remain and some alternative solution will need to be devised to deal with them. This new solution, whatever it is, will likely come under attack from those who pushed for ObamaCare.

Lost in the contentious debate about healthcare is the general agreement over the main problems that need to be addressed in order to fix the current system. These are so big that they are impossible for anyone to ignore and as such they are a good starting point to understand what ObamaCare is all about.

ObamaCare Attempts to Fix Big Problems

So what exactly are the main problems that ObamaCare sought to fix when it was being drafted a few years ago? The official title of the new law — the Patient Protection and Affordable Care Act — gives us a general idea of what the authors of the legislation intended. Broadly speaking, they had four main goals in mind:

1. **Give Americans greater access to healthcare** — As of today, about 37 million American citizens have no health insurance at all, in many cases because it's simply too expensive for them to buy. The new law opens the door to the healthcare system for these uninsured Americans and ushers them inside with financial assistance so that they can get basic coverage, either through Medicaid (the program will be dramatically expanded) or subsidized health insurance via exchanges (which will be set up in each state or, for those states who don't create their own programs, the federal government).

2. **Rein in (and ideally reduce) out of control healthcare costs** — Americans certainly love their healthcare, but it comes at a high price, with spending per person in the United States at a level well above the amount spent in most other developed countries. Exploding medical costs are a big and growing problem, not only making it more difficult for all of us to afford health insurance, but also weakening the entire nation as rapidly rising expenditures on entitlement programs like Medicare and Medicaid threaten to bankrupt the country in future decades. ObamaCare accordingly attempts to "bend the cost curve" down and reduce the amount of money the United States spends on healthcare, mainly by encouraging a movement away from the current fee-for-service system, which critics say drives up costs because it rewards doctors for increasing the quantity of their care (e.g., encourages them to perform often-unnecessary tests and procedures) rather than quality.

3. **Add more consumer benefits and protections** — Although healthcare in the United States is generally considered the best in the world (assuming you have access to it), getting decent care can be difficult for many Americans. ObamaCare removes glaring inequities from the current system by creating an impressive bulwark of new consumer safeguards and benefits. It prevents insurance companies, for example, from dropping your coverage after you get sick because you made a minor error when you filled out your application. And thanks to ObamaCare, they can no longer refuse to extend you coverage because you have a pre-existing health condition or charge you a higher premium because you're older or have a chronic disease that increases your use of healthcare. Coverage can no longer have annual or lifetime limits.

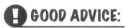 **GOOD ADVICE:**

ObamaCare...prevents insurance companies from dropping your coverage after you get sick because you made a minor error when you filled out your application. And thanks to ObamaCare, they can no longer refuse to give you coverage because you have a pre-existing health condition or charge you a higher premium because you're older or have a chronic disease that increases your use of healthcare.

4. **Address a host of other nagging issues** — The new law also includes a smorgasbord of provisions intended to reach different goals, most of which are praiseworthy but difficult to achieve. In one section it strives to make Americans healthier by emphasizing prevention and wellness programs. Another part provides more help for those who need assisted-living, long-term care (as mentioned, this component of ObamaCare called CLASS has been officially suspended by the White House). And there is an array of pilot programs to test new ways of delivering and paying for healthcare with the goal of improving efficiency and reducing cost in the system.

Before we explain in full how ObamaCare goes about trying to reach these major goals, here's a snapshot of how the new law will affect ordinary Americans and major stakeholders in the healthcare system. We'll follow up this summary of the law's impact by running through the timetable for the rollout of ObamaCare's biggest components.

OBAMACARE: WHAT IT MEANS FOR YOU

2

WHAT DOES OBAMACARE MEAN FOR YOU? That depends on who you are, the conditions of your life, your financial status and the extent of your involvement in the healthcare industry. Here are the key groups most affected by the new law:

The Insured

ObamaCare is a mixed-bag for those who currently have health insurance. On the plus side, the law adds a host of new consumer benefits and protections. The question, of course, is the impact these new "goodies" will have on the amount you have to pay for your coverage. Even more worrisome, if you have insurance through your employer, there is a chance that your coverage will be dropped because of rising prices. Other negatives: The penalty for making non-allowable purchases from Health Savings Accounts will increase to 20 percent, and the amount of money your employer can contribute to your Flexible Spending Account will be capped at $2,500. If you are on Medicare, your benefits will shrink thanks to ObamaCare's spending cuts, which will discourage some plans and care providers from serving Medicare beneficiaries. If you are on Medicaid, the program could be overwhelmed by the millions of new enrollees, eroding the quality of care you receive right now.

The Uninsured

If you have no health insurance right now, ObamaCare is, on the whole, great news for you. If you have a low income, you will either be able to enroll in Medicaid or qualify for a subsidized insurance plan through your state's healthcare exchange (or, if your state doesn't run one, the federal government's). If you have a high income, you will also be able to buy a plan through an exchange, and its price will probably be better than what you would have to pay on the private insurance market today. That's because you won't be an isolated buyer, but rather a member of the large group made up of all those who are purchasing through the exchange.

Senior Citizens

If anyone wonders whether ObamaCare is good for seniors, all they need to do is look at the results of the 2010 congressional elections; voters age 65 and over voted for Republicans by a large majority (59 percent to 38 percent according to the exit polls). Seniors were rightly angry about ObamaCare as it is significantly funded with money that comes from hundreds of billions of dollars in spending cuts to Medicare over the next decade. It also cuts benefits in the Medicare Advantage program. When the bill was signed into law in 2010, budget forecasters projected those cuts would total $455 billion over the next decade. Since then, the Congressional Budget Office has twice updated that figure to reflect new realities. In 2011, the CBO estimated ObamaCare would cut Medicare by $507 billion between 2012 and 2021. Then in July 2012, the CBO projected Medicare outlays would be reduced by about $716 billion between 2013 and 2022. On the plus side for seniors, ObamaCare expands Medicare's prescription drug coverage and coverage for certain preventive care services. It also caps what insurers can charge older Americans for premiums because of their age. But this is small consolation and does little to offset the broader punishment it inflicts on the Medicare program as a whole. And even more painful, spending cuts may be on the horizon as the law creates a powerful new panel called the Independent Payment Advisory Board, which will be given unprecedented control over Medicare's budget in a few years.

Taxpayers

Broadly speaking, taxpayers will be hurt by ObamaCare as about half of its funding comes from new taxes and fees imposed directly and indirectly on Americans – amounting to more than $400 billion over the next decade. One tax is of particular concern since it goes into effect on January 1, 2013, and threatens to affect homeowners. This is the new 3.8 percent ObamaCare surtax on capital gains above $250,000 (married couples). If you are worried about the financial impact of this tax if you decide to sell your home, remember that President Clinton signed a special homeowners' exemption to the capital gains tax in the 1990s and it remains in place, neutralizing the ObamaCare tax in most cases. Under that exemption a married couple is not taxed on any capital gains up to $500,000 on the sale of the home they live in. They pay a 15 percent tax on all profits above this level and with the ObamaCare surtax added the amount rises to 18.5 percent.

The Affluent

ObamaCare is not good news for the highest-earning Americans as they will be asked to pay much more to help fund the healthcare of the rest of the population. Single Americans who earn above $200,000 per year (or $250,000 for couples) will see the amount they pay in taxes for Medicare

> **? DID YOU KNOW . . .**
> ObamaCare is a mixed-bag for those who currently have health insurance. On the plus side, the law adds a host of new consumer benefits and protections. The question, of course, is the impact these new "goodies" will have on the amount you have to pay for your coverage.

hospital insurance increase from the current 1.45 percent level to 2.35 percent above those income thresholds. Medicare beneficiaries with higher income will also be required to pay higher Part D premiums. A heavy 40 percent tax will also be imposed above a specific threshold level for premiums on so-called "Cadillac" health insurance plans that some big earners now enjoy (see Appendix A). While few people have extravagant plans like these, it's a big tax increase nonetheless considering the rate goes from zero abruptly all the way up to 40 percent.

Working Families

With health insurance premiums rising since ObamaCare was passed in 2010, middle-class families have thus far found no relief from the heavy healthcare expenses they carried on their shoulders before then. The new consumer protections and benefits provided by ObamaCare will help families, but they come at a cost that insurers will pass onto ordinary Americans in the form of higher premiums. Beyond this expense, the degree to which ObamaCare helps or hurts families will depend upon income levels. Those that fell between the cracks of the old system – that is to say, those which earned too much to qualify for Medicaid but earned too little to afford private insurance – will likely be helped when subsidized health insurance plans become available on the state-based exchanges which begin operating in 2014.

The Poor

In most states, Americans with the lowest incomes are big winners under ObamaCare. Under the new law the income requirement to get into Medicaid is raised to 133 percent of the federal poverty line. Unlike Medicare, which generally provides healthcare for Americans 65 years of age or older, Medicaid is chiefly designed to help the poor and disabled below that age. It is jointly run by the federal government and the states. If fully implemented, an estimated 15 million more people will be able to get coverage as a result of the ACA, and low-income earners who still can't get into Medicaid will in most cases qualify for generous government subsidies offered on the new state exchanges. Having said this, the actual expansion of Medicaid will probably fall short (at least in the near term) of the 15 million new enrollees predicted. The Supreme Court has ruled that states cannot be penalized if they refuse to increase the number of Medicaid enrollees within their borders, and a handful of states with Republican governors, like Texas and Florida, have announced that they will not go along with the plan.

The Unemployed

If you're unemployed and actively looking for work, ObamaCare has, in many instances, already hurt your chances of finding a job. According to the Heritage Foundation, job creation in the private sector stalled in April 2010 right after the law was passed and has not recovered since that time. The massive stimulus that injected almost a trillion dollars into the economy right after President Obama took office added some government-sector jobs and lowered the nation's unemployment rate somewhat. But businesses continue to be reluctant to hire new workers in part because each hire now costs significantly more due to ObamaCare mandates that many companies must provide for their employees' healthcare or pay a penalty. Some have argued that repealing ObamaCare would generate a huge job surge.

Children Under Age 18

The youngest Americans have not been affected much by ObamaCare and their open access to healthcare will continue into the future. As a last resort, healthcare coverage is already guaranteed to children under the Medicaid program. This will not change, but now private insurance plans will no longer be able to reject children because they have a pre-existing health condition (a provision that extends to adults in 2014).

Young Adults Age 18 to 29

Although 20-somethings voted for President Obama by a two-to-one margin over John McCain in the 2008 election, ObamaCare is nothing less than a grab at their wallets and purses. The individual mandate is largely targeted at the young and healthy, and is used to strong-arm them into paying for something most of them don't want. All young Americans with libertarian leanings who place a premium on personal choice were undoubtedly disappointed when the Supreme Court upheld the constitutionality of the individual mandate. It will likely end up costing young Americans a few thousand dollars a year in new health insurance expenses or a similar amount in the form of a significant fine payable to the Internal Revenue Service. On the plus side, many more young people will have health insurance if ObamaCare becomes fully operational.

Illegal Aliens

Those residing in the United States without proper documentation proving they are here legally will not be able to access any of the new benefits that come with ObamaCare. They will not be able to buy health insurance through the new state-operated exchanges, nor will they be allowed into the Medicaid or Medicare programs. Because illegal aliens are officially considered outside the system, they will also not have to comply with the individual mandate. Although illegal aliens have no official right to health insurance, they are still entitled to care through hospital emergency rooms, which according to law cannot deny treatment to any individual regardless of citizenship status. In an effort to help them further, ObamaCare has increased funding to the often overlooked 1,200 community health centers in the country, which many illegal immigrants rely upon.

Groups Singled Out by ObamaCare

Right now, older Americans pay more for health insurance than younger citizens, tobacco users pay more than those who abstain and residents in high cost-of-living areas pay more than those who live in less-expensive regions of the nation. Under ObamaCare, price discrimination by insurers among these groups will be allowed to continue, but the amount they can charge will be capped. For example, older Americans will never have to pay more than three times the amount for their health insurance than younger citizens. Adult children up to age 26 will now be eligible for coverage under a parent's health plan as long as that plan includes coverage for dependent children.

Large Businesses

From a cost perspective, ObamaCare has thus far not been good for large companies as new mandates imposed on their health insurance providers have increased business operating costs. The new healthcare exchanges, however, could eventually bring these rising costs under control and provide employers with more options when they seek to purchase insurance for their workers. While large businesses wait and hope for this positive outcome, many have had to resort to non-compliance waivers issued by the Department of Health and Human Services to sidestep the sudden increase in their operating costs. Ultimately, many large businesses may decide to drop health insurance coverage for their workers altogether and instead pay a $2,000 fine per worker if they decide it is in their financial interest to do so.

Those Who Work for a Large Business

Many Americans are worried that ObamaCare will force their employer to drop their insurance. This is a legitimate fear, but less so if you work for a big business. Most large businesses would probably prefer to drop coverage and pay the $2,000 fine per worker (it is much less than what premiums cost), but many see health insurance benefits of vital importance to compete effectively in the labor market. If they dropped their coverage, they might lose many valuable employees. If you work for a large business like McDonald's, which does not pay well and which does not need a health insurance carrot to attract workers, you are in greater danger of losing your coverage.

Small Businesses

The ObamaCare legislation effectively defines a company with 25 or fewer employees as a "small business." Such companies are hurt by rising healthcare costs just as much as their larger corporate siblings, but they will benefit more from ObamaCare in the short term. That's because of significant tax breaks they will receive against the amount they pay in health insurance premiums for their workers. Small businesses will also have immediate access to health insurance plans sold through the exchanges beginning in 2014 while large businesses will have to wait for this privilege, assuming it is granted to them at all (each state will have to decide for itself whether or not to let large businesses purchase insurance through its exchange). Small businesses have historically had to pay significantly more than large businesses to insure their workers, not only in premiums, but also in administrative costs. The new ObamaCare health exchanges promise to create more of a level playing field and, if they succeed, small businesses could realize large financial benefits. Again, it is important to note that ObamaCare's assistance for small business accrues only to companies with 25 or fewer employees. If a small business exceeds that number, it will receive no tax credits from the IRS.

Those Who Work for a Small Business

On the whole, ObamaCare is great news for those employed by small businesses. Most currently do not provide health insurance for their workers and now will be encouraged to do so with a generous tax credit. If they pass on this benefit, workers will be able to buy insurance through a government-subsidized exchange, probably at a below-market price. With an exchange-based insurance plan, workers are not anchored to a single company and are thus free to switch jobs or work as a freelancer without losing coverage. There are also provisions for individuals purchasing coverage through an exchange to earn tax credits.

Unions

It's good to be in a labor union if you don't like ObamaCare. Of the 1,625-plus non-compliance waivers granted thus far by the White House, more than half have gone to protect union workers. That's about two million union workers who have benefited. This group, which represents many of President Obama's most ardent supporters, has been singled out for temporary immunity from the costly effects of the new law. As with the waivers granted to businesses, it remains to be seen what will happen when the waivers obtained by labor unions expire in 2014. They could be extended. If they're not and health insurance costs have not by then been brought under control, union workers will be forced to pay more along with the rest of the nation's labor force.

Doctors

While ObamaCare has angered a significant portion of the American people (especially seniors), the anger among doctors is palpably strong. In a poll conducted in 2010 for the Physicians Foundation, 40 percent said they would "retire, seek a non-clinical job in healthcare or seek a job unrelated to healthcare" during the next three years. Fears of an acute doctor shortage, which existed prior to ObamaCare, have only been exacerbated by the new law. The anger of doctors is understandable as ObamaCare reduces their earning potential by, for instance, putting new restraints on payment rates in Medicare. In a larger sense, the law represents an ideological assault on the current fee-for-service system – the foundation of most doctors' earnings. New payment systems like Accountable Care Organizations (ACOs) might not hurt doctors financially, but there is a big risk they will, leaving them with lower incomes to pay off medical school student loan debts that are among the highest in the world.

> **? DID YOU KNOW . . .**
>
> In a poll conducted in 2010 for the Physicians Foundation, 40% of doctors said they would "retire, seek a non-clinical job in healthcare or seek a job unrelated to healthcare" during the next three years.

Patients

It's a good bet that ObamaCare will degrade, on average, the level of care patients receive today. Millions of more doctor visits will occur in the United States each year with as many as 30 million additional people now enjoying the benefits of health insurance coverage. This flood of new patients will likely water down care for everyone. But the problem may be made worse because doctors are now under new pressure to cut back on their services, to limit the number of tests they do and so forth. ObamaCare's ultimate goal is to replace the current fee-for-service system with Accountable Care Organizations (ACOs), which some critics believe are simply a repackaging of Health Maintenance Organizations (HMOs), which developed a notorious reputation for denying certain types of care to patients strictly out of financial considerations.

Healthcare Professionals

If you work as a nurse in a hospital, an accountant for a health insurance provider or in any other job in the healthcare field, ObamaCare is good and bad news. All the changes that come with the new law will inevitably make your job more difficult, but on the other hand your job is probably more secure than ever. The demand for healthcare professionals is likely to rise significantly in coming years with so many more Americans carrying insurance. The complexities of ObamaCare are daunting for ordinary citizens, which means those who have expert knowledge of its intricacies will probably enjoy a salary advantage on the labor market. So your salary could rise, too.

Nursing Homes

CLASS, the centerpiece of ObamaCare's long-term care solution, was shelved by the White House after it could not prove itself financially stable. This insurance plan was designed to keep more seniors at home during the last lap of their lives, saving the expense and other downsides that come with residence in a nursing home. CLASS's demise is good news for the nursing home industry since its population of residents is now not likely to decrease. As for residents themselves, they will be protected by new regulations that, for instance, require that nursing home ownership is transparent and that states monitor the conditions of facilities more closely. These are designed to improve the quality of life for residents, but it remains uncertain whether their impact will be positive.

Insurance Companies

One might think that insurers would be unhappy about ObamaCare because of the new rules it imposes upon them, but they supported the law and hailed its passage. It's easy to see why, as it will provide them with about 30 million more customers (assuming every state eventually expands Medicaid), many of whom will have their insurance bill paid for by the federal government. The individual mandate will also deliver more paying customers and businesses to insurers. That's not a bad deal for insurers, especially when one considers that they are free to pass on the higher costs from ObamaCare mandates to their customers. In case you forgot, that's you and me.

Drug Companies

Like the insurance industry, Big Pharma (the Pharmaceutical Research and Manufacturing Association) also benefits from a massively expanded market for the drugs companies manufacture. Its support for ObamaCare was so strong that it even agreed to provide billions of dollars in subsidies to expand Medicare's prescription plan and close its infamous "donut hole," which is a large coverage gap that has been in place since Medicare started paying for prescriptions for seniors during the Bush Administration. Pharmaceutical firms will also have to offer some expanded discounts (rebates) to Medicaid.

OBAMACARE: A MULTIYEAR TIMETABLE

3

I F YOU FEEL OVERWHELMED by the complicated rollout of ObamaCare, you're not alone. To help keep track of the important dates, here is the law's basic timetable, including an accounting of the parts of the law that have already taken effect.

As for the dates to come, keep in mind that these could change as a result of political actions, changes in Washington and other factors. The White House, of course, could also change its planned implementation dates for ObamaCare components if it so chooses, as it did when it suspended the CLASS long-term care insurance program.

Implementation Dates

March 2010	President Obama signs the Patient Protection and Affordable Care Act into law.
July 2010	Government-run "high-risk pool" set up to provide insurance for adults with a pre-existing

health condition until all insurance plans provide this coverage in January 2014.

September 2010   Children under age 18 can no longer be rejected by insurers because they have a pre-existing health condition.

Children up to age 26 can be insured as dependents covered by their parents' insurance policy.

Insurance plans can no longer impose a lifetime limit on a policyholder's benefits.

Insurance plans can no longer impose an annual limit on a policyholder's benefits (phase-in begins with total ban effective January 2014).

Insurance companies can no longer use "rescissions" to abruptly cancel policies for frivolous reasons.

Maximum tax credit of 35 percent available to small businesses with 25 or fewer employees.

January 2011   "Donut hole" in Medicare's prescription drug plan begins to close (it disappears completely by 2020).

Health Savings Account and Flexible Spending Account funds can no longer be used to pay for over-the-counter drugs.

October 2012	Enrollments in CLASS long-term, assisted-living care insurance program were to begin (Note: CLASS was suspended by the White House in October 2011).

January 2013	Income tax deduction threshold for medical expenses rises from 7.5 percent of income to 10 percent.

January 2014   Medicaid expanded across the United States to an income level up to 133 percent of the federal poverty line in every state (a handful of states, including Texas and Florida, have announced that they will not go along with this part of ObamaCare and because of the Supreme Court ruling the federal government cannot punish them financially for their non-compliance).

Health exchanges selling insurance to individuals and small businesses begin to operate in each state in the United States (if a state does not set one up — some like Florida and Alaska have announced they won't — the federal government will create and run it for them).

Individual Mandate Tax — Americans who do not obtain health insurance expose themselves to a maximum penalty of $285 per year.

Adults age 18 and older can no longer be rejected for

GOOD ADVICE:

Parents should know: Children under age 18 can no longer be rejected by insurers because they have a pre-existing health condition. Children up to age 26 can be insured as dependents covered by their parents' insurance policy.

insurance because of a pre-existing health condition. Young adults under age 30 can buy low-priced catastrophic insurance through the exchanges.

Insurance plans must cover "essential health benefits" (approved preventive tests covered as of September 2010).

Maximum tax credit of 50 percent available to small businesses with 25 or fewer employees (available for two years before it expires at the end of 2015).

January 2015 **Individual Mandate Tax** — Americans who do not obtain health insurance expose themselves to a maximum penalty of $975.

Independent Payment Advisory Board (IPAB) can begin making recommendations to cut Medicare spending.

January 2016 **Individual Mandate Tax** — Americans who do not obtain health insurance expose themselves to a maximum penalty of $2,085.

January 2017 Health exchanges can be opened to large businesses with more than 100 employees if a state chooses to let them in.

October 2017 Earliest date CLASS long-term, assisted-living care insurance benefits were to be paid out (Note: CLASS was suspended by the White House in October 2011).

January 2018 Independent Payment Advisory Board's recommendations about Medicare's budget can be implemented.

Tax on "Cadillac" insurance plans (40 percent on the value of a plan above specific thresholds) begins (see Appendix A).

HEALTH INSURANCE: RADICAL CHANGES AHEAD

4

To UNDERSTAND OBAMACARE it is important to put it in the context of what was in place before its arrival on our doorsteps. When we look at the pre-ObamaCare healthcare system, what do we see? One thing immediately catches our attention. Healthcare in the United States has traditionally been delivered and paid for in a very different manner than that seen in most developed countries in the world.

Much of the world relies, in large part, on socialized medicine to take care of its citizens. The United States, in contrast, uses a mixed system which combines elements of socialized medicine (through government-subsidized programs like Medicaid and Medicare) with employer-based healthcare (where the employer and employee share the cost of health insurance).

The employer-based system traces its roots to Chancellor Otto Von Bismarck, who unified Germany in the 1870s and created the modern welfare state. About 70 years later, Bismarck's employer/employee cost-sharing scheme took hold in the United States during World War II when the American government imposed wage controls to prevent salary inflation as millions of men suddenly left the labor force and were enlisted to fight Germany and Japan.

Looking for a way — besides direct wages — to reward workers, businesses began to offer healthcare benefits to their employees. Since that time, employer-based health insurance has come to dominate and define the American healthcare system, in part because benefits are provided to employees on a tax-free basis. This aspect of the system has proven advantageous, but it also inadvertently created a glaring inequity because it excluded self-employed individuals, who get no tax break when they buy health insurance on their own using after-tax dollars.

Other deficiencies of the employer-based system have not gone unnoticed. Critics make a persuasive case that it encourages overuse of healthcare. Because employees don't directly pay for their benefits, they simply use them as if they were free, not appreciating their real value. Using the logic that if you tax something you will inevitably get less of it, many experts insist that the way to hold down healthcare costs is to tax employee healthcare benefits.

Today Most (But Not All) Americans Get Help Buying Health Insurance

What does the nation's healthcare system look like as it pertains to different parts of the population? Let's break the system down into the important groups, highlighting how much financial help each gets with their healthcare.

In 2010 roughly 150 million Americans (that's 48 percent of the population) received their health insurance with a big helping hand from their employer, which on average contributed the lion's share (about 70-80 percent) of their employees' premiums. While the employer contribution in many cases results in reduced wages for the employee, it is still a financial benefit that the uninsured and self-employed do not enjoy.

A sizeable portion of the remaining population (28 percent) also gets help obtaining healthcare. These are needy Americans — the elderly, poor and disabled — who receive government financial assistance for coverage in the form of Medicare (15 percent of the population) or Medicaid (13 percent).

Added together, those with employer-based insurance and those in government programs like Medicare and Medicaid amount to 76 percent of Americans, all of whom receive financial assistance for their healthcare. Most of the remaining 24 percent of the population are uninsured or buy individual healthcare coverage on the insurance market. Simply put, Americans in this group are at a distinct disadvantage compared to the rest of the country when it comes to healthcare.

TAB. 4-1: HEALTH INSURANCE IN THE UNITED STATES BY GROUP (2010)			
	People	Share	Most Recipients
Medicare	47	15%	Retirees & Disabled
Employer Insurance	150	48%	Low to High Income
Private Insurance/Other	27	9%	Medium to High Income
Uninsured*	50	16%	Young Adults, Low Income
Medicaid/CHIP	40	13%	Poor & Children
Total People (Millions)	314	100% up to 101%	

*Includes illegal aliens and Medicaid eligibles who have not signed up.
Source: Congressional Budget Office

Helping Those Who Need the Most Help

ObamaCare will affect all Americans to some degree, but it's mainly targeted at the one in four Americans who today receive no financial help if they try to obtain health insurance. Let's take a closer look at the two large sub-groups among them:

- Those In The Private Insurance Market — Making up about 9 percent of the population, these Americans are financially able to buy insurance

? DID YOU KNOW . . .

In 2010 roughly 150 million Americans (that's 48% of the population) received their health insurance with a big helping hand from their employer, which on average contributed the lion's share (about 70-80%) of their employees' premiums.

on their own but typically have to pay significantly higher insurance premiums, co-pays and deductibles than everyone else. That's because they must use after-tax dollars to make their purchase (those who buy through their employer use pre-tax dollars). They are at an additional disadvantage because they are single, stand-alone buyers unable to leverage the purchasing power of a large group such as a big corporation, a union or the government, each of which has the size and clout to negotiate lower prices for their insurance plan enrollees. Although it is not yet apparent, the new law should eventually help lower prices in the private insurance market by giving its members the chance to buy insurance at reasonable prices in a newly created health insurance exchange in each state. Moreover, those with low enough incomes will be able to get a government subsidy to help reduce the price they pay when they buy through an exchange. Tax credits will also be extended for purchasing coverage.

② DID YOU KNOW . . .

As of 2010 the uninsured represent about 16% of the population of the United States (about 50 million people in total).

- **The Uninsured** — As of 2010 the uninsured represent about 16 percent of the population of the United States (about 50 million people in total). A big chunk of this group are illegal aliens (about 13 million people), who work off the books for the lowest wages. The rest are American citizens (about 37 million people) who fall through the cracks of the current system. Many of these are young adults who enjoy robust health, while others are low-income people under age 65 (that's when eligibility for Medicare begins) whose work circumstances don't give them easy access to employer-based healthcare and who simultaneously make too much money to qualify for Medicaid. ObamaCare will help provide affordable healthcare coverage for most uninsured citizens by simply buying all or most of it for them, either through Medicaid (which will be dramatically expanded) or in new health insurance exchanges (which will be heavily subsidized to reduce prices). Another group within the uninsured that will benefit from the ACA are those individuals who could not purchase health insurance due to significant illness histories or pre-existing conditions. Insurance plans will no longer be permitted to deny offering coverage to these formerly "medically uninsurable" people.

While ObamaCare sets out to insure as many Americans as possible, it does not guarantee universal healthcare coverage throughout the United States. Most forecasts predict that coverage will reach about 95 percent of the population under the new law — an increase of roughly 11 percentage points above the current 84 percent level. If big states like Texas and Florida, however, follow through on their intention not to expand Medicaid as envisioned by the law, the coverage level could fall short of the 95 percent expectation.

Of those who remain uninsured after ObamaCare goes into full operation, most will be illegal aliens (who will remain ineligible for Medicaid and will not be allowed to buy insurance through the exchanges) in addition to a relatively small group of Americans who refuse to comply with the individual mandate requiring them to get health insurance or pay a fine. These uninsured individuals will still be able to use hospital emergency rooms and community health centers to receive care. Some of the medically uninsurable group may also remain uninsured if they find insurance now available, but not necessarily affordable.

ObamaCare's Impact on Different Groups

ObamaCare offers both good news and bad news for specific groups of Americans. Here's a breakdown of how it will impact key individuals:

MEDICARE RECIPIENTS

For those who currently receive Medicare benefits, ObamaCare is on the whole a bitter pill to swallow. It includes one significant improvement that senior citizens will applaud, but more importantly singles Medicare out and makes it a special target for spending cuts.

Good News

- The infamous "donut hole" in Medicare's prescription drug coverage will finally close. No longer will seniors spend a few thousand dollars on prescription drugs only to discover that Medicare no longer covers the cost of drugs unless they spend a few thousand more. Under ObamaCare, recipients will have robust prescription drug coverage regardless of how much they spend. Keep in mind, however, that the "donut hole" will be slowly phased out over the next decade and won't completely close until 2020.

Bad News

- Like most of us, many seniors are wondering who is going to pay for ObamaCare. If you're a Medicare recipient, the answer is you. According to the Congressional Budget Office, hundreds of billions of dollars in funding for ObamaCare will be generated by cuts in Medicare's budget over the next decade.

- The biggest spending cuts will come in two areas: reduced number of plans available and reduced benefits in the Medicare Advantage program (which allows enrollees to use private insurance to supplement their basic Medicare coverage), and reduced payment rates to doctors who care for Medicare patients.

President Obama and Congressional Democrats have promised that the cuts to Medicare will not adversely affect the quality of care seniors have come to expect, but at this point that is only their expectation, not a guarantee.

If doctors, hospitals, and other providers react negatively when they are paid less, some may refuse to see Medicare patients, making it more difficult for some to find a doctor or see the one they're accustomed to using. If you are part of Medicare Advantage, some of your benefits, such as gym memberships and vision care, might disappear.

Perhaps more troubling for seniors is the way ObamaCare emphasizes the need to control Medicare's costs further down the road. The law creates a new presidential commission called the Independent Payment Advisory Board or IPAB (think of it as the U.S. Federal Reserve Board for healthcare rather than banking). This board will be given significant power to cut Medicare spending in the future because its decisions will automatically take effect unless counteracted by Congress. That will be hard to do as it will require a three-fifths "super-majority" vote in the U.S. Senate.

The driving idea behind the IPAB is to give political protection to the president and members of Congress by allowing unelected government officials ("healthcare commissars" might be the best way to describe them) to make the toughest budgetary decisions. Because these officials won't have to stand for election before the American people they will, in theory, be able to cut Medicare's budget in a way that is not possible today.

If the operations of the IPAB seem undemocratic to your ears, you're not alone. It has many harsh critics, and its survival is very much an open question. Republicans in Congress have promised to take aim at the IPAB.

But unless ObamaCare is changed, there is no getting around the

! GOOD ADVICE:

Under ObamaCare, insurers won't be able to place lifetime limits on your benefits. Check with your employer to see if you are affected by any of the new provisions. You should expect at least minor changes in your coverage.

ax that is wielded by the current law. ObamaCare explicitly cuts into Medicare's budget and also includes a ticking time bomb in the form of the IPAB, which if not defused, will mean even more spending cuts in the future. How might these be executed? ObamaCare includes a number of pilot programs to test new ways to manage Medicare through innovations such as Accountable Care Organizations (ACOs) and other "bundled payment" schemes (discussed later in this book). If pilots like this work on a small scale, the IPAB could decide to expand them to the whole country.

INDIVIDUALS WITH EMPLOYER-BASED INSURANCE

If you're covered under an employer's healthcare plan, ObamaCare has probably already hurt you as premiums and deductibles have gone up for most working families since the law's passage. Even worse pain could be on the way if you happen to work for a company that decides your health insurance is too expensive under new ObamaCare mandates and decides to drop your coverage altogether.

Good News

- New rules and regulations will likely improve certain aspects of your employer-based coverage. For example, under ObamaCare, insurers won't be able to place annual or lifetime limits on your benefits. Check with your employer to see if you are affected by any of the new provisions. You should expect at least minor changes in your coverage.

- Small businesses will likely benefit from the new health insurance exchanges once they begin to operate in 2014. These exchanges will offer standardized healthcare plans at prices that will be the best on the market. Initially, large companies will not have access to the exchanges, but beginning in 2017 each state, if it chooses, will be able to let companies of all sizes use them.

Bad News

- Small employers like McDonald's, which provide barebones, low-cost health insurance (called "Mini-Meds" in industry jargon) to their workers, have already come close to dropping their coverage because of the heavy financial burden of new ObamaCare mandates. If you work for one of these companies, your coverage could be threatened if your employer hasn't been able to obtain a non-compliance waiver which allows them to sidestep the law. Without a "get out of jail free" waiver, some large employers will undoubtedly decide to drop health insurance coverage for their workers, especially those that do not need such benefits to attract workers. If they do, they will have to pay a $2,000 fine per worker, but that could save them money compared to paying health benefits since most employers pay much more in premiums per worker. How many businesses will drop coverage for their workers? Hard to say. The consulting firm McKinsey and Co. thinks it could be as high as 30 percent, while Deloitte Consulting Services says it will only be 10 percent.

INDIVIDUALS WITH PRIVATE HEALTH INSURANCE

If you're self-employed or in another circumstance that forces you to buy health insurance on your own, you could eventually be helped by ObamaCare.

Good News

- The new law was created in part to help level the playing field for those forced to buy expensive health insurance as self-employed individuals, compared to those who have easy access to the lower prices that come with an employer-based plan. Under ObamaCare, individual buyers will have access to affordable plans sold through health insurance exchanges, where they'll be able to buy at the prices everyone else on the exchange pays. And if an individual's income is low enough, he or she will be able to qualify for a government subsidy to help reduce the amount paid.

- Individuals in the private health insurance market have not only had to deal with higher premiums, their coverage has usually come with onerous requirements and fewer protections than those offered in the employer-based group market. ObamaCare again comes to the aid of these self-employed buyers by allowing them to purchase insurance that comes with the same protections that employer-based plans enjoy.

Bad News

- Healthcare costs in the United States have risen since ObamaCare's passage, affecting all types of insurance, whether it is employer-based or found in the private insurance market. If the current trend persists, premiums, co-pays, and deductibles will continue to go up for individual policyholders, just like everyone else's.

THE UNINSURED

ObamaCare was created first and foremost to help the uninsured, so if you fall into this category, the law naturally is good for you. But, there are some who will not applaud the new law because it will force them to buy a service they do not want. These individuals, however, are likely to represent a relatively small minority of the uninsured.

Good News

- Like those in the private health insurance market, uninsured individuals will now have access to the health insurance exchange in their home states. If you fall into this category, these exchanges will offer a selection of different healthcare plans, and if your income is low enough, you will be able to get a subsidy to lower the price you pay when you buy a plan.

- If your income is really low, you will now qualify for Medicaid which, under ObamaCare, will be significantly expanded by raising the income threshold to 133 percent of the federal poverty line. As a result, millions more Americans will be able to sign up for the program and you could be among them. Some states have announced that they will not participate in Medicaid's expansion, so if you are a resident of one of these, it will be more difficult for you to enroll in the program. But if you can't, you will be able to buy subsidized insurance on the state's health exchange.

Bad News

- For those among the uninsured who do not qualify for Medicaid or a subsidy on the health insurance exchanges (those with incomes above 400 percent of the federal poverty line will not receive financial assistance from the government), ObamaCare could cost you money. That's because the individual mandate included in the new law forces you to get insurance or pay a fine.

- Many young and healthy Americans will not like ObamaCare for this reason. This sub-group of the uninsured — those who don't have health insurance as a matter of choice — will no longer be able to stand outside the system and pay nothing into it, using their own bank account or a hospital emergency room as a fall-back for medical assistance in a time of need.

By 2019 ObamaCare is expected to reduce the number of uninsured Americans from 41 million (if the law had not been created) to about 10 million — a 75 percent reduction in the number of uninsured citizens. That's a dramatic improvement compared to how things stand today. It will come at an immense price, of course, which ultimately will be passed on to the American consumer purchasing health insurance and the taxpayer, who will face a barrage of new taxes and levies.

MEDICAID/CHIP

If you currently receive Medicaid or CHIP (the Children's Health Insurance Program), you're likely to be the group least affected by ObamaCare, but there are a few things to watch out for.

Good News

- One of the biggest problems with Medicaid today is that many doctors refuse to see Medicaid patients because of the program's relatively low payment rates. ObamaCare tries to fix this problem by raising Medicaid reimbursement rates to Medicare levels, and thus you may see an increase in the number of doctors who will take you as a patient (Note: The rate increase only applies to primary care doctors, not specialists). This assumes that higher payment rates will be sufficient to offset other financial pressures that doctors may be forced to bear under ObamaCare, which simultaneously reduces their payment rates for Medicare patients. If a doctor shortage occurs because of the new law, that will, of course, diminish or negate this potential benefit as well.

Bad News

- Because about 15 million more people are expected to enroll in Medicaid as the program is expanded over the next decade (assuming all states eventually agree to participate) there is a possibility that the system could be overwhelmed. One of the reasons ObamaCare is being phased in over a number of years is to give everyone involved time to prepare. Each state will need to put resources in place to deal with millions of new people coming into the program beginning in 2014. It's one reason why so many states have reacted negatively to ObamaCare and why 26 of them mounted a legal challenge against it.

- If you live in a state like Massachusetts or Minnesota that currently has generous eligibility requirements, you might actually be pushed out of the Medicaid program. If you are enrolled in Medicaid right now in one of these states and your income is above 133 percent of the federal poverty line, beginning in 2014 you will no longer be eligible for the program. Instead you will be forced to buy subsidized insurance through your state's health exchange. It probably will not cost you much with the financial assistance you will be given by the government, but it will be more than what you were paying to be in Medicaid, which comes free of charge to recipients.

The ObamaCare Scorecard: Winners and Losers

The biggest winners under ObamaCare are obviously the uninsured, who will now get basic coverage that provides "essential health benefits" at a relatively low cost (in some cases they will pay nothing out-of-pocket). Another winner: Those in the private health insurance market will now be able to buy insurance with the same advantages that employer-based plans enjoy.

Other groups will likely see less positive effects. Even if a number of states refuse to expand Medicaid, the program could be overwhelmed by the millions of new recipients who will flow into it. Some doctors already are reluctant to treat Medicaid patients and their resistance could grow.

Employer-based plans will benefit from more consumer protections. Somewhat ominously, however, they will be taxed for the first time to raise money to fund ObamaCare and to suppress what the architects of the new law believe has been the excessive healthcare usage associated with the "Cadillac" tier of coverage (see Appendix A). Some big businesses may also decide to drop employee coverage and instead pay a $2,000 per worker fine to the government.

The biggest losers under ObamaCare are Medicare recipients. Senior citizens are thrown a bone with the closure of the "donut hole" in the program's prescription drug plan, but that will not offset the hundreds of billions of dollars in budget cuts over the next decade. And once the Independent Payment Advisory Board (IPAB) begins to operate, additional cuts seem likely.

TAB. 4-2: **WHO BENEFITS MOST/LEAST FROM OBAMACARE?**	
Biggest Winner	**Comments**
Uninsured	Finally Get Covered at Low/No Cost
Private Insurance Market	Lower Prices/New Protections
Medicaid/CHIP Recipients	System Could Be Overwhelmed
Employer-Based Plans	Taxed for First Time, Could Drop Coverage
Medicare Recipients	$455 Billion in Spending Cuts
Biggest Loser	

Some groups will obviously benefit from ObamaCare more than others, but if the new law eventually proves successful and improves the healthcare system of the United States by decreasing the number of uninsured, providing more consumer protections while simultaneously holding down healthcare costs, all Americans should be pleased.

On the other hand, if the new law continues to drive up the price of our premiums, co-pays, and deductibles, and in the process creates another ravenous, budget-busting entitlement monster, we will have good reason to be unhappy with ObamaCare.

PART II
INSURING THE UNINSURED

"The Supreme Court upheld the constitutionality of the individual mandate and defined it as a 'tax.' But whether it's called a tax, a penalty or a fine, it means only one thing: non-participation in ObamaCare will cost you financially."

THE INDIVIDUAL MANDATE 5

W HEN THE AUTHORS OF OBAMACARE sat down to craft legislation that would reform and improve the healthcare system of the United States they had one goal that took precedence over all others: reduce the number of uninsured Americans as much as possible.

They had good reason to focus their attention on this group, as it has grown at an alarming rate in recent years. In 2000 about 38 million Americans were uninsured. With the recent economic downturn that number had spiked to 50 million by 2010 — a 32 percent increase compared to a decade ago.

Making the problem even worse during this time, employers grew increasingly reluctant in light of the steady rise in healthcare costs to offer health insurance to their employees. Add this all up and more than 20 percent of the working age population (those under age 65) count themselves today among the uninsured.

To understand the overwhelming emphasis that ObamaCare puts on filling in this gaping hole in the nation's healthcare system, all we need to do is follow the money. When we do, we discover that a massive 84 percent share of ObamaCare spending — or $899 billion — goes toward decreasing the uninsured population over the next decade.

This is the amount needed to pay for the expansion of Medicaid (assuming all states participate) and the new state-based health insurance exchanges. In comparison, the rest of the money to be spent under the new law ($176 billion) seems almost like an afterthought. Given these budgetary facts, it would not be unreasonable to describe ObamaCare as simply "Healthcare for the Uninsured."

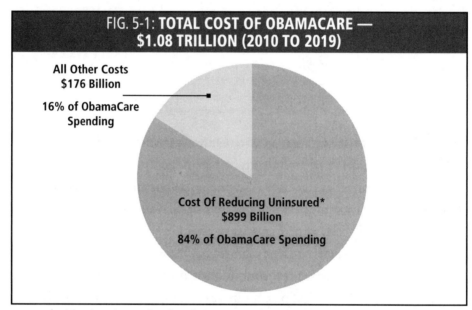

FIG. 5-1: **TOTAL COST OF OBAMACARE — $1.08 TRILLION (2010 TO 2019)**

All Other Costs
$176 Billion

16% of ObamaCare Spending

Cost Of Reducing Uninsured*
$899 Billion

84% of ObamaCare Spending

*Combined cost of Medicaid expansion and new health insurance exchanges.

IMPACT OF SUPREME COURT RULING ON MEDICAID EXPANSION

Empowered by the Supreme Court's ruling, a handful of states have indicated that they will not be participating in the expansion of Medicaid. Right now, it is impossible to predict how many of them will ultimately stay on the sidelines, making it difficult to know the number of new Medicaid enrollees after 2014. Because of this, we have reverted back to the original Congressional Budget Office estimate of 15 million more enrollees, which assumes that every state will participate. The CBO believes that the non-participation of a few states in the short term will reduce the cost of ObamaCare by about $84 billion — a rough estimate.

One factor the authors of ObamaCare had to consider: why so many do not have health insurance. As it turns out, the uninsured remain outside the current system for a variety of reasons, but mostly as a matter of personal choice or because of poor financial circumstances.

Many believe:

- **Health Insurance Is Not Necessary** — Enjoying robust health, millions of Americans live for today, not tomorrow, oblivious to the possibility that a sudden illness or accident could wipe out their financial resources in the blink of an eye. This mindset is particularly true of young adults, who are often referred to as "invincibles" by health insurance professionals.

- **Health Insurance Is Too Expensive** — If you're young and healthy, you might be reluctant to buy health insurance even at a very low price, but there are many Americans who would get coverage if they were financially able to do so. This sub-group among the uninsured lives just above the poverty line. Unable to participate in an employer-based plan or qualify for Medicaid, they fall through the cracks of the current system.

Perceiving the reality that many healthy Americans would not want to pay for health insurance even at a bargain-basement price, President Obama and Congressional Democrats saw that they would need to do more than simply make health insurance affordable. They would also need a coercive stick.

The Massachusetts example — the new healthcare system it created in 2006 that is the model for ObamaCare — revealed the importance of an individual mandate. A handful of states had tried universal coverage before, but all failed because people were free to opt out. Massachusetts was the first to put an individual mandate in place and it worked like a charm, increasing the number of insured in the state to 97 percent — the highest level of any state in the country.

Learning an important lesson from Massachusetts' success, the authors of ObamaCare focused on pushing "invincibles" into the system because those who are young and healthy inevitably need much less healthcare than others. Their financial contributions would thus help subsidize health insurance for all Americans because they would put in more than they take out, at least in the short term. That balance, insurance companies argued, would help pay the increased costs for expanding coverage for the poor and those who pay less but use more healthcare resources (such as seniors and those with chronic or pre-existing conditions).

Knowing that under current law any citizen could refuse to buy health insurance, the law's supporters understood that there was only one way to achieve their objective: They must use the force of law to compel universal participation. And so, out of necessity, ObamaCare includes what is perhaps its most controversial component, the individual mandate.

Simply put, it makes it a legal requirement for all Americans to get healthcare coverage and penalizes them financially if they do not. Under this government decree healthy, Americans will have to pay into the system for their own good whether they like it or not. The Supreme Court upheld the constitutionality of the individual mandate and defined it as a "tax." But whether it's called a tax, a penalty or a fine, it means only one thing: non-participation in ObamaCare will cost you financially unless you can somehow wriggle out of its grasp.

Although the individual mandate is nothing less than a libertarian's nightmare — the nanny state on steroids deciding that it must take care of its citizens because they cannot or will not take care of themselves — it wasn't put into the new law on a tyrannical whim. In truth, it is an indispensible piece of ObamaCare, a keystone that enables and supports the rest of the law's goals and initiatives.

Is the Individual Mandate Really Necessary?

President Obama and his party knew that the individual mandate would generate stiff public resistance, but they included it in the final law anyway for a host of reasons. Among them:

STRENGTHEN THE NATION'S HEALTH INSURANCE "RISK POOL"

The viability of any type of insurance depends in large part on its ability to spread risk across as many people as possible. By adding as many as 30 million of the uninsured (most of them young and healthy) into the healthcare system, the nation's insurance "risk pool" is dramatically strengthened. A large influx of healthy Americans (the group with the lowest risk) creates a much more balanced system than the current one.

> **? DID YOU KNOW . . .**
> Massachusetts was the first to put an individual mandate in place and it worked like a charm, increasing the number of insured in the state to 97% — the highest level of any state in the country.

PRE-EXISTING CONDITION REJECTIONS

One of the most important parts of ObamaCare is the provision that prevents insurance companies from rejecting people because they have a pre-existing health condition. Under this provision, all Americans are guaranteed coverage regardless of their health status. While this is a wonderful new consumer benefit, it also strongly encourages people to refuse to pay premiums and stay uninsured, confident that they can get coverage whenever they want. The only way to overcome this obstacle — to make sure no one can take advantage of the government's guarantee and sit on the sidelines until they need care — was to force everyone to make financial contributions before the fact.

OFFSET INCREASED COSTS FROM OTHER OBAMACARE RULES

The ObamaCare provision that prevents insurance companies from rejecting adults because of a pre-existing health condition will undoubtedly raise insurance costs as will others. The most important of these provisions prevents insurance companies from placing a limit on the amount of annual or lifetime benefits that a beneficiary can receive. The individual mandate makes all of these new rules possible because it guarantees insurance companies as many as 30 million more customers to offset the new financial burdens they must shoulder as a consequence.

DEFER TO A POLITICAL NECESSITY

The need for an individual mandate was also driven by a stark political reality. In the 1990s the health insurance industry was among the fiercest opponents of the healthcare reform legislation proposed by President Bill Clinton. If industry leaders were not placated this time around, ObamaCare would have had little chance of getting through Congress. The individual mandate proved to be an effective enticement to get insurance companies on board as a significantly increased market proved irresistible to them. Not only will they have millions of more buyers of their insurance policies, the government will give the new customers money to make their purchases.

While the insurance industry struck a deal with President Obama and Congressional Democrats to secure passage of the new law, it made no promises about the prices insurers would charge American consumers for health coverage in the post-ObamaCare world. The new ObamaCare rules and their associated costs have already compelled insurance companies to pass these costs onto their customers through higher premiums, co-pays, and deductibles, all of which have risen since the law was passed. There is no reason to believe this troublesome trend will stop, especially when one considers that even more ObamaCare mandates hit insurers beginning in 2014. Insurers, doctor practices, hospital systems, and healthcare providers are all looking for ways to control costs by pushing preventive care, outpatient programs, and other initiatives. But ObamaCare does not require those efforts or provide many market incentives to drive down costs, so the impact they will have remains uncertain.

First the Stick, Then Some Carrots

The individual mandate is unquestionably a coercive stick, but ObamaCare also includes a few carrots that lessen the pain of its heavy-handed directive. The carrots come in the form of government financial assistance to help low-income Americans obtain health insurance (either through Medicaid or an exchange) and tax credits that give small businesses a financial incentive to offer health insurance to their employees.

For Americans who have low incomes, the individual mandate will be far from oppressive as they'll be given healthcare (i.e., something of significant value) either for free or at a price well below what they would have to pay in today's private insurance market. Small businesses will also be helped through the tax credits. These will prove less beneficial than the help individuals receive, however, as they'll last only six years (2010 to 2015). Let's take a closer look at each carrot in turn.

The first one is straightforward enough. Under ObamaCare, the doors of Medicaid will be thrown wide open and millions of Americans will now qualify for the program. That's because the income threshold to qualify for Medicaid will be raised in 2014 to 133 percent of the federal poverty line ($29,327 for a family of four in 2010) in most states in the country.

We say "most states" because some have signaled their intention not to participate in Medicaid's expansion. The original ObamaCare law said that if a state stayed on the sidelines, it could lose all of the federal dollars that helps pay for Medicaid within its borders (right now, Washington pays on average 57 percent of Medicaid's cost in each state). But the Supreme Court has now ruled that this coercive financial stick is unconstitutional, empowering states to keep their Medicaid enrollment at current levels without losing millions of federal dollars if they choose to do so.

Prior to the new law, each state could set its own income threshold for entrance into the program at or above a certain floor level, and many states choose to let only a bare minimum of people into Medicaid. ObamaCare tried to strip this power from the states and make it the exclusive domain of lawmakers in Washington. It's one reason why 26 states filed a lawsuit over the issue, complaining that this element of the law was a violation of their state's sovereignty as guaranteed by the 10th Amendment to the Constitution. The Supreme Court ultimately agreed with them, ruling that the federal government did not legally possess this coercive power.

The states won the right to maintain their current Medicaid enrollment levels if they choose, but there are generous financial subsidies still in place that will pay for about 93 percent of the cost of so-called "new eligibles" through the year 2020 in those states that agree to participate. This is a powerful financial incentive considering the 57 percent level of federal funding in place right now for current Medicaid enrollees.

While resistance to ObamaCare's expansion of Medicaid is strong right now in some states, it will probably fade with so much money offered from Washington. According to the Congressional Budget Office, if all states ultimately agree to participate, the expansion of Medicaid will decrease the uninsured population by 15 million people by 2019.

Government financial assistance to obtain health insurance is not limited to increasing Medicaid enrollment. It will also be available for the new state-based health insurance exchanges, with the amount of the subsidy available to individuals depending on where someone's income falls on a sliding scale relative to the federal poverty level.

The exchanges, which will begin operating in 2014 just as Medicaid expands, will provide subsidized insurance coverage to all those who fail to qualify for Medicaid and who earn below 400 percent of the federal poverty line ($88,200 for a family of four in 2010). The subsidized exchanges are projected to decrease the number of uninsured by 16 million people by 2019.

Standing side by side like imposing entitlement pillars, the expansion of Medicaid and the new exchanges raise the edifice of ObamaCare up off the ground, creating a gigantic new infrastructure that will shelter more than 30 million of the newly insured under its remarkably broad and expensive umbrella.

TAB. 5-1: **IMPACT OF OBAMACARE ON UNINSURED (2019)**		
	Without ObamaCare	**With ObamaCare**
Uninsured*	41 Million	10 Million
		+
Now Insured		31 Million
(Insured by Medicaid Expansion**)		(15 Million)
(Insured by Healthcare Exchanges)		(16 Million)
		=
Total Americans	41 Million	41 Million

*Excludes 13 million illegal aliens not eligible for new government aid
**Assumes all 50 states participate in Medicaid expansion
Source: Congressional Budget Office

Who Will Be Able to Get Government Financial Assistance?

Eligibility for Medicaid or subsidies for an exchange plan will depend on which state a person lives in. If a person is a resident of a state that has chosen not to participate in ObamaCare's expansion of Medicaid, the following rules will not apply. But for those who live in states that have agreed to participate (most experts believe 40 or more will go along with the plan), eligibility requirements for Medicaid enrollment will be significantly loosened, with higher income individuals now being let into the program.

Here's how it will work from top to bottom within the income range established by the new law. Those with

? DID YOU KNOW . . .

New state-based health insurance exchanges will begin operating in 2014 to provide subsidized insurance coverage to individuals who fail to qualify for Medicaid or Medicare or are not covered through employer-based healthcare plans.

an income up to 133 percent of the federal poverty line (or $29,327 for a family of four in 2010) will be eligible for Medicaid. Those with an income between 133 percent and 400 percent of the poverty line ($88,200 for a family of four in 2010) will be able to get financial assistance from the government to buy healthcare coverage on their state's exchange.

TAB. 5-2: **ELIGIBILITY FOR GOVERNMENT ASSISTANCE (UNDER AGE 65)***			
Family of 4 Income Level	**Percent of Poverty Level***	**Individuals Can Get Coverage In:**	**Government Subsidies?**
Above $88,200	Above 400%	Their State's Health Exchange	No
$88,200	400%	Their State's Health Exchange	Yes
$29,327 $22,050** $0	133% 100% 0%	Medicaid	Yes

*Applies only in those states that have agreed to ObamaCare's expansion of Medicaid
**Federal poverty level in 2010 (Source: Dept. of Health & Human Services)

Those with an income above 400 percent of the poverty line will still be able to buy coverage through their state's exchange, but they'll be ineligible for government financial assistance. Although they will be out of luck in this regard, the price of health insurance plans through the exchanges should, in theory, be lower than anything they could find today on the private insurance market. In this sense, the exchanges should benefit all Americans seeking to obtain coverage on their own.

ObamaCare also includes a third, less direct carrot to help Americans obtain health insurance by incentivizing small businesses to offer health insurance to their employees. If these employers offer their workers a basic level of coverage, they will qualify for tax credits. Large businesses will be pushed in the opposite direction; if they do not offer their employees basic coverage, they will have to pay financial penalties.

Supreme Court Ruling on the Individual Mandate

Supporters of the individual mandate argue that coercive insurance mandates are not new in the United States. They point out that every American who wants to drive an automobile must first obtain car insurance. Critics of the individual mandate answer that this is a flawed analogy because driving is considered a privilege, not a natural right, and a citizen chooses to own a car, which sparks the requirement for insurance. They also note that Americans can opt out of buying car insurance simply by not owning a car — a non-participation option is not available under ObamaCare.

Although it seems unprecedented for the government to force Americans to buy a particular service or product, there are many examples of government compelling its citizens to behave in certain ways for their own health and safety. The law requiring drivers to wear seat belts is just one example.

Whatever one may think about the merits of the individual mandate, the issue has been decided for us by the highest judicial body in the land, which sidestepped all of the complicated arguments for and against it. The Supreme Court ruled in June 2012 that the mandate was simply another "tax" and thus constitutional under the federal government's long established power to tax Americans.

It was a controversial ruling, especially since the word "tax" is not found in the language of the law itself, and because the Obama administration denied that the individual mandate was a "tax," calling it a "penalty." As much as we may scratch our heads over these odd aspects of the court's ruling, the bottom line is that the individual mandate is here to stay. Only an amendment to the Constitution could strike it down now and that is highly unlikely.

Penalties for Not Obtaining Health Insurance

If you're worried about being criminally prosecuted and put in jail for not getting health insurance under ObamaCare, don't be. The law specifically states that this will not happen. It also says that the government cannot put a lien on your property as a means to pressure you to obtain health insurance if you adamantly refuse to do so.

The law, however, does empower the Internal Revenue Service to seize tax refunds as payment toward an unpaid penalty. This power is significant as almost half of all income tax returns processed by the IRS result in a refund to the taxpayer. The average refund in 2011 was about $2,700, which means that in most cases it will be big enough to pay the individual mandate penalty.

> ❓ **DID YOU KNOW . . .**
>
> **The individual mandate takes effect in 2014 and if you don't obtain health insurance that year, you will have to pay either a flat fee of $95 or 1% of your income up to a maximum of $285 (the amount of the fine is capped at triple the flat fee).**

About half of all taxpayers will therefore be in danger of the IRS seizing their income tax return if they don't comply with the individual mandate, but all Americans could be menaced in another way. The IRS is free to write intimidating letters, threatening jail and large financial penalties for non-compliance to any citizen, regardless of whether they receive an income tax refund or not. This power should not be underestimated, as many fear the IRS almost as much as the Grim Reaper. As Elizabeth Maresca of the Tax & Consumer Litigation Clinic put it, "Most people pay because they're scared and I don't think that's going to change."

How much will the fine be if you do in fact have to pay it? The amount will vary depending on the year it's incurred. The individual mandate takes effect in 2014 and if you don't obtain health insurance that year, you will have to pay either a flat fee of $95 or 1 percent of your income up to a maximum of $285 (the amount of the fine is capped at triple the flat fee). You will have to pay whichever amount is higher in your case.

After that, the penalty will grow until it reaches a ceiling in 2016 — a flat fee of $695 or 2.5 percent of your income up to a maximum of $2,085. As in previous years, you will have to pay whichever amount is higher for you.

TAB. 5-3: **PENALTY FOR NOT OBTAINING HEALTH INSURANCE**					
Year	Flat Fee: Amount		Percent of Income: Level	Maximum**	Income Level
2014	$95	or*	1.0%	$285	$28,500
2015	$325	or*	2.0%	$975	$48,750
2016	$695	or*	2.5%	$2,085	$83,400
After 2016	Adjusted For Cost of Living				

*Those without insurance must pay whichever of these sums is greater
**The maximum penalty is fixed at 3 times the flat fee

Who Will Be Hurt Most by the Individual Mandate?

Keep in mind that only a small fraction of Americans will have to worry about the individual mandate and the financial penalty that comes with it. If you already have health insurance (that's 84 of every 100 of us), you won't have to pay any penalty since your existing coverage means that you comply with the law.

Of the 37 million who were uninsured in 2010 (not counting 13 million illegal aliens), about 14 million will be able to obtain healthcare coverage without paying anything out of their own pocket by enrolling in Medicaid after its expansion. This group of people can avoid the penalty by simply signing their name on a piece of paper. Another 14 million currently uninsured Americans will be able to receive government financial assistance when they buy coverage through their state's exchange. With this help, it will probably be less expensive for many in this group to buy subsidized insurance than to pay the fine.

TAB. 5-4: **VULNERABILITY TO "INDIVIDUAL MANDATE" PENALTY**		
Key Sub-Groups	Total In 2010	Percent of U.S. Population
Uninsured Americans in 2010 (Total People)	**37 Million***	**12%**
Covered by Medicaid Expansion**	**14 Million**	**4.5%**
Can buy through Exchanges (with subsidy)	**14 Million**	**4.5%**
Can Buy through Exchanges (without subsidy)	**9 Million**	**3%**

*Excludes 13 million illegal aliens
**Assumes all 50 states participate in ObamaCare's expansion of Medicaid

The remaining group of uninsured (about 9 million Americans or 3 percent of the population in 2010) will also be able to buy coverage through the exchanges, but they will have to do so without a subsidy. This is the group of Americans with the greatest financial incentive to refuse to comply with the individual mandate. Although this is only a sliver of the total population, in absolute terms 9 million is not a small number of people.

While the coercive aspect of the individual mandate ruffles the sensibilities of many Americans who feel an oppressive government breathing down their necks, the pain of its imposition is lessened considerably by the expansion of Medicaid and the subsidized healthcare exchanges.

There are also select groups of people who will be exempt from any financial penalties if they do not get health insurance. These include:

- Those who can prove a financial hardship (i.e., the lowest cost plan they could obtain through their state's exchange is greater than 8 percent of their income)

- Those who have an income below the tax filing threshold ($9,350 for individuals and $18,700 for joint filers in 2010)

- Native Americans (who receive health insurance in a separate government program)

- Those who have been without health insurance for only a brief time (3 months or less)

- The prison population

- Those with religious objections

- Illegal immigrants (they will not be subject to a financial penalty because they don't have health insurance, nor will they be able to buy health insurance on the exchanges)

It should be noted that young adults up to the age of 26 can also escape the individual mandate penalty by remaining a dependent covered by their parents' health insurance. This provision of ObamaCare took effect in September 2010.

Young adults under age 30 have another option. They will be able to buy a "catastrophic health plan" through their state's exchange at a price below that of the least expensive plan available for adults age 30 and older (the so-called "Bronze" plan sold on each exchange, which covers 60 percent of medical costs on average).

While staying on their parents' insurance plan or buying a catastrophic plan provides young adults alternatives to the extremes of either buying full health insurance coverage or refusing to get any coverage at all, these alternatives also undermine the overall strength of ObamaCare. The new healthcare system will be weakened significantly if the young and healthy "invincibles" are allowed to escape making financial contributions into the new system as their participation is needed to strengthen the insurance "risk pool" for all Americans.

How Will I Prove That I Have Health Insurance?

The IRS has yet to announce guidelines, but it has made indications that proving health insurance coverage will probably follow the current procedure which is used to report investment income to the government. If your employer provides your health insurance, the company will likely be required to provide paperwork to the IRS stating that fact. The same procedure would apply if you hold a private insurance policy, except your insurer would have to report your coverage. If you happen to have coverage through Medicaid, Medicare or on a state's health exchange, that fact will automatically be reported to the IRS.

GOOD ADVICE:

If you're a young adult, you should investigate whether you can remain on your parents' health insurance plan (those under age 26 qualify). Also, young adults under age 30 will have another option in 2014: They will be able to buy a "catastrophic health plan" through their state's exchange at a price below that of the least expensive plan available.

THE EXPANSION OF MEDICAID 6

IN ITS EFFORT TO decrease the number of uninsured Americans, ObamaCare wields a coercive stick called the individual mandate, making it a legal requirement for every American to get health insurance or pay a fine. It then offers up three carrots that help soften the blow: the expansion of Medicaid, the creation of health insurance exchanges and financial incentives for small businesses. In this chapter we focus on Medicaid's expansion. In the chapters that follow we discuss the other carrots in turn.

TAB. 6-1: MEDICAID EXPANSION — MANDATE & GOVERNMENT ASSISTANCE			
The Stick	**The Individual Mandate**		
	Every one has to get health insurance or pay fine		
	↓	↓	↓
The Carrots	**Government Assistance in the Form of ...**		
	Medicaid Expansion	Exchanges	Small Businesses
	Fully Subsidized	Partially Subsidized (on Sliding Scale)	Tax Credits (on Sliding Scale)

To appreciate the scope of the Medicaid expansion planned under ObamaCare, let's step back and look at Medicaid as it exists today. Created in 1965, the Medicaid program provides health insurance for the poorest Americans and children who would otherwise have none. It's managed jointly by the states and the federal government, with each paying a share of the costs. The states run the program on a day-to-day basis, but the federal government controls how it functions and determines (with some important limits on its power) who can enroll.

Who is eligible for Medicaid today? The chart below summarizes the core federal eligibility requirements for the program, expressed as a percentage of the federal poverty level for individual households. States must let people into the program who have incomes that fall below these minimum levels.

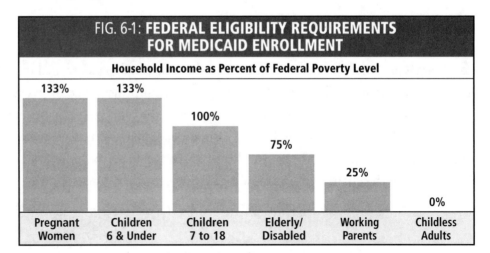

Pregnant women and young children can enroll in Medicaid if their household income level is below 133 percent of the federal poverty line. The threshold drops to 100 percent FPL for school-age children. The elderly and disabled also may enroll, but the threshold is again lower (75 percent FPL). For working parents it drops all the way down to 25 percent FPL. As of mid-2012, the federal government does not require that the states let childless adults into the program.

Keep in mind these are the minimum federal eligibility thresholds. States can and often do increase them so more citizens can enroll in Medicaid. In some cases they receive federal matching funds for letting more people in, but in others they are on their own and must pay the full amount for the coverage of the extra people they let in.

ObamaCare's intention was to set the income threshold for all these groups at 133 percent of the federal poverty level, including childless adults. That is why 26 states filed a lawsuit against the law, with the Supreme Court eventually ruling in their favor, saying that the federal government could not put "a gun to the head" of the states and force them to increase Medicaid enrollment in this way. The court said the decision to expand enrollment was up to the states, not Washington.

The Supreme Court's decision regarding Medicaid's expansion, which significantly weakens but does not kill ObamaCare, was applauded by critics of the law, including many Republican governors. Chris Christie of New Jersey was pleased, telling a receptive audience at the Brookings Institution: "I was glad that the Supreme Court ruled that extortion is still illegal. That's a relief. Because ObamaCare on Medicaid to the states was extortion. It essentially said you expand your program to where we tell you, and if you don't, we're taking all the rest of your money away."

> **"Medicaid is a system of inflexible mandates, one-size-fits-all requirements and wasteful bureaucratic inefficiencies."**

Believing that the sovereignty of individual states needs to be respected more than it currently is, Governor Rick Perry of Texas was just as happy to have more flexibility to manage Medicaid without Washington's interference. He went further than Christie, blasting the weakness of the Medicaid program itself and blaming its deficiencies on decades of mismanagement by the federal government.

"Medicaid is a system of inflexible mandates, one-size-fits-all requirements and wasteful bureaucratic inefficiencies," wrote Perry in a letter to Health and Human Services Secretary Kathleen Sebelius. Later he told Fox News: "Medicaid is a failed program. To expand this program is not unlike adding a thousand people to the Titanic."

As colorful as that metaphor is, history suggests Medicaid will survive. All the evidence we have of the life cycle of big federal entitlement programs is that they continue to grow and suck up more taxpayer dollars. Enjoying special political protection because so many voters rely on the benefits they provide, none of them have thus far disappeared and Medicaid is a long way from sinking under its own weight, with the federal government standing ready to keep it afloat even as it takes on water.

The Current Medicaid Landscape: An Uneven Playing Field

Because of flexibility in the law, some states allow more people into Medicaid than they are required to by the federal government, while others take a harder line and maintain narrow eligibility requirements, restricting the number of enrollees to a select few.

> **"Medicaid is a failed program. To expand this program is not unlike adding a thousand people to the Titanic."**
> – Governor Rick Perry of Texas

A person's eligibility for Medicaid therefore depends very much on where he or she lives as shown in Table 6-2, which singles out six states based on the variance in their average Medicaid eligibility requirements. The numbers you see are the income thresholds for states ranked #1, #11, #21, #31, #41 and #51 (the District of Columbia is included in the ranking), expressed as an index to the federal poverty level (275 = 275 percent above the line).

TAB. 6-2: **PRE-OBAMACARE MEDICAID INCOME THRESHOLDS** **(% OF FEDERAL POVERTY LEVEL)**									
State	Jobless Parents	Working Parents	Children's Age			Pregnant Women	Adults w/o Children	Avg	Rank*
			0-1	1-5	6-19				
Minnesota	275	275	280	275	275	275	Not Eligible	276	1
N. Mexico	30	69	235	235	235	235	Not Eligible	173	11
Tennessee	73	134	185	133	100	250	Not Eligible	146	21
Kentucky	36	62	185	150	150	185	Not Eligible	128	31
S. Dakota	54	54	140	140	140	133	Not Eligible	110	41
Alabama	11	25	133	133	100	133	Not Eligible	89	51

*Fifty states and District of Columbia
Source: Kaiser Family Foundation

If you're a working parent and want to get Medicaid coverage today, your greatest chance of success is in Minnesota, where the income threshold is the highest in the United States. Put another way, Minnesota — with its average income threshold at 275 percent of the federal poverty level — lets a bigger share of its working parent population into Medicaid than any other state in the country.

What does this mean in 2010 dollars? Working parents in Minnesota can receive Medicaid benefits if their income is below $60,638 (which is equal to 275 percent of the poverty level for a family of four). This is far more generous than Alabama, where working parents can receive Medicaid benefits only if their income is below $5,513 (which is equal to 25 percent of the poverty level). Minnesota's door into Medicaid is thus a startling 11 times more open to working parents than is Alabama's.

ObamaCare Levels the Playing Field

Under ObamaCare, the confusing, inconsistent, and arguably unfair mishmash of Medicaid income eligibility levels across the nation disappears and is replaced by a single standard, at least for those states that agree to participate in the law's planned expansion of the program.

As we've discussed, the Supreme Court in June 2012 struck down an important coercive provision of ObamaCare which said that if a state decided not to expand the number of Medicaid enrollees as the law required, then it would risk losing all of its federal support for the program.

With this part of the law now null and void, states are free to reject ObamaCare's expansion of Medicaid without losing any of their federal support. A large amount of money was at stake as Washington paid on average 57 percent of the cost of Medicaid in each state.

At the time this book went to press it was still not clear how many states would agree to participate in the expansion of Medicaid, but as many as 10 could decide to opt out. Texas, Florida, Mississippi, Virginia and South Carolina have already indicated they are leaning toward non-participation and others, especially those with Republican governors, may join them.

For the 40 or more states who do decide to increase their Medicaid rolls under ObamaCare's auspices, the expansion will set the Medicaid enrollment threshold at 133 percent of the federal poverty level for all groups, raising the current level for school-age children from 100 percent FPL, the elderly/disabled from 75 percent FPL and working parents from 25 percent FPL. Childless adults, who the federal government said could be left out of the program altogether in the past, now must receive full admittance as long as their income is below 133 percent FPL.

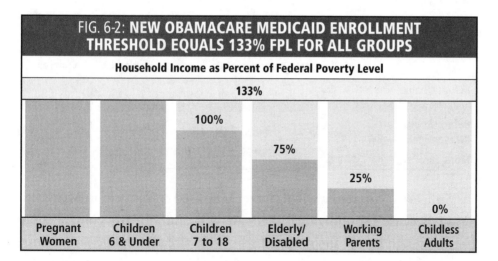

FIG. 6-2: **NEW OBAMACARE MEDICAID ENROLLMENT THRESHOLD EQUALS 133% FPL FOR ALL GROUPS**

Household Income as Percent of Federal Poverty Level

133%

100%

75%

25%

0%

| Pregnant Women | Children 6 & Under | Children 7 to 18 | Elderly/ Disabled | Working Parents | Childless Adults |

What does this mean? For one thing, there will no longer be any differences in eligibility requirements between two states like Minnesota and Alabama, both which will now have the same income threshold for all Americans under age 65 (senior citizens, of course, will continue to primarily rely on Medicare for their health insurance).

How will Americans be able to find out whether they qualify for Medicaid under the new rules? That will be easy. All they will have to do is contact their state's health insurance exchange, which will be tasked with determining every American's eligibility for government assistance, whether for Medicaid or for subsidies to help buy insurance through an exchange.

Medicaid Expansion Will Affect Each State Differently

The impact of ObamaCare on each state will depend in large part on what the state's Medicaid income eligibility levels were before the new legislation was passed. For instance, Minnesota will be affected less than many other states because its annual income thresholds are already more than double those that will be required by ObamaCare.

TAB. 6-3: **IMPACT OF MEDICAID EXPANSION ON MINNESOTA**							
	Jobless Parents	Working Parents	Children's Age			Pregnant Women	Adults w/o Children
			0-1	2-5	6-19		
Before ObamaCare (Minnesota's threshold)	275	275	280	275	275	275	**Not Eligible**
Before ObamaCare (New minimum level)	133	133	133	133	133	133	133
More Enrollees?	Probably a Slight Increase						Yes

Still, even Minnesota will likely see increased enrollment in Medicaid. Why? Because the individual mandate will undoubtedly compel some people to sign up for the program who were already eligible but did not enroll, whether out of ignorance or indifference.

Enrollment will also dramatically increase because of those who are now for the first time permitted to enroll in Medicaid, even in a state like Minnesota, which already has very loose eligibility requirements. Like every other state, it will now have a flood of adults without children signing up for Medicaid benefits. New enrollees will come into Medicaid across the country because of this provision, again assuming the state agrees to participate in ObamaCare's expansion of the program.

At the other end of the impact spectrum is Alabama, which will be affected by ObamaCare more than any other state if it agrees to participate in the expansion. Medicaid enrollment in this state will likely increase for the same reasons it will increase in Minnesota, but in Alabama there is a much bigger factor at play. Because its Medicaid income eligibility levels are currently very narrow, enrollment in the program will dramatically increase under ObamaCare.

TAB. 6-4: **IMPACT OF MEDICAID EXPANSION ON ALABAMA**						
	Jobless Parents	Working Parents	Children's Age			Pregnant Women	Adults w/o Children
			0-1	1-5	6-19		
Before ObamaCare (Alabama's threshold)	11	25	133	133	100	133	Not Eligible
Before ObamaCare (New minimum level)	133	133	133	133	133	133	133
More Enrollees?	Big Increase		Slight Increase				Yes

Prior to ObamaCare, a working parent in Alabama had to make less than $5,513 (25 percent of the poverty level) to qualify for Medicaid. When Medicaid is expanded in 2014, the same working parent could make as much as $29,327 (133 percent of the poverty line for a family of four) and still get in. That's almost a six-fold increase in the income eligibility level.

Minnesota and Alabama are polar opposites used here to illustrate the impact of ObamaCare on the states. All states that agree to participate will be affected by Medicaid's expansion to some degree that falls between these extreme cases and some will obviously benefit more than others in terms of decreasing the number of uninsured within their borders.

We've talked at length about all the new people who will be eligible for Medicaid. Ironically, some of the program's current enrollees will actually lose their eligibility under ObamaCare. For instance, people currently in Minnesota's Medicaid program who earn above the 133 percent federal poverty line will be forced to move to the state's health exchange. When they do, they will receive a generous federal subsidy to buy their insurance, but their new coverage will cost them some money out-of-pocket and this amount, whatever it is, will be higher than what they pay for Medicaid, which is free to its enrollees.

Who Pays for Medicaid's Expansion?

According to the Congressional Budget Office roughly 15 million more people will sign up for Medicaid by 2019 as a result of ObamaCare. This estimate assumes the participation of all 50 states in the country plus the District of Columbia. After the Supreme Court ruling, states are now free to opt out of the expansion of Medicaid without incurring a financial penalty. Because of this, some states will not participate, but the exact number that will opt out is unknown.

> **"With more people on Medicaid, states will have to continue to ratchet down payments and limit services."**
> — Nina Owcharenko, an expert on health policy at the Heritage Foundation.

Whether the number of new Medicaid enrollees is 15 million or something lower (the actual expansion will probably fall 10-20 percent below this prediction for the whole country), who will pay to provide healthcare for all of these people? Most of it will be funded by the federal government, with individual states eventually contributing a small share to cover new people entering the program.

States like Alabama (assuming it agrees to participate in the expansion) that had income thresholds in Medicaid far below 133 percent of the poverty level before ObamaCare will benefit most from the federal funding. A huge swath of the uninsured in this state will finally get healthcare coverage and the federal government (in other words, the American taxpayer) will pay nearly all of the Medicaid costs of these newly insured. Not a bad deal if you live on a low income in Alabama.

Here's how it will work: When the doors to Medicaid open wide in 2014, all of the new people who sign up above the federal government's old income thresholds will be classified as "newly eligible." The federal government will pay to cover these newcomers according to the following phased-in payment schedule:

TAB. 6-5: **PAYING FOR NEW MEDICAID ENROLLEES UNDER OBAMACARE***		
Year	**U.S. Government**	**Each State Pays:**
2014 to 2016	100%	0%
2017	95%	5%
2018	94%	6%
2019	93%	7%
2020	90%	10%

*Applies only to states that agree to participate in Medicaid's expansion
*Includes Medicaid eligibles who have not applied

In the first three years of ObamaCare, the federal government will pay for 100 percent of all the "newly eligible" people in Medicaid, with the level reduced to 90 percent by 2020. These levels of financial support for the states are much higher than the current contribution the federal government makes to each state to support Medicaid. As it currently stands, the states only get between 50-75 percent of their Medicaid costs covered by the federal government (levels vary based on a state's wealth). Today, on average, the federal government picks up 57 percent of the cost of Medicaid for each state.

Against this established standard, the increased funding for Medicaid under ObamaCare is a great deal for the states, at least in the short term. But states like Texas and Florida are leaning toward not participating in the program's expansion out of worry that the large federal contribution will drop significantly after 2020, creating a ticking time bomb that might eventually blow up their already strained budgets. Right now, there are no guarantees in the law that the ObamaCare level of federal support for "new eligibles" will be maintained, so in this sense the fear is reasonable.

States considering opting out of Medicaid's expansion are also worried about a flood of so-called "old eligibles" to the program. These are the many individuals who could have signed up for Medicaid without ObamaCare's eligibility changes, but did not do so out of indifference or ignorance. The financial burden for states from these "old eligibles" will be heavier than for "new eligibles" since the federal government will pay for them under the old formula, which covers only 57 percent of their cost on average.

How many "old eligibles" will sign up to Medicaid? A scholarly article in the *New England Journal of Medicine* by Ben Sommers and Arnold Epstein estimates that only 62 percent of those eligible for Medicaid today have actually enrolled in the program. In Texas and Florida the participation rates are even lower, at 44 percent and 48 percent respectively. The authors of the analysis estimate that nine million Americans across the country are currently not receiving Medicaid, but could if they would simply sign up for it.

It's anyone's guess how many of these nine million will sign up for Medicaid because of ObamaCare, but if about half do that will mean four or five million more enrollees for the states to absorb — enrollees that will only have 57 percent of their cost funded from Washington and not the 93 percent funding amount promised for "new eligibles."

Governors like Perry and Scott have good reason to worry about Medicaid expansion. Some states like California have already expanded the programs, permitting new people to come in under the new ObamaCare eligibility thresholds that take effect in 2014. It has added 400,000 uninsured residents to its Medicaid program, a level it expects to rise to 500,000 within two years.

This is a generous policy, but it is made in a state where Medicaid reimbursement rates to doctors ranks 47th out of 50 states in the country. The door for new enrollees is wide open in California, but the quality of its program is hurt by shifting the financial burden onto the shoulders of doctors, many of whom simply refuse to see Medicaid patients. When doctors are shortchanged, Medicaid patients are ultimately hurt because they have difficulty finding a doctor who will care for them and, if they are fortunate enough to find one, often experience lengthy waiting times and have to travel long distances to get the care they need.

As Nina Owcharenko, an expert on health policy at the Heritage

Foundation, put it: "With more people on Medicaid, states will have to continue to ratchet down payments and limit services." Seeing this problem the federal government has increased payment rates to primary care doctors who take Medicaid patients to the higher Medicare level, but the increase is only temporary and will expire at the end of 2014.

Seen in this light, the expansion of Medicaid will not be smooth sailing. It will increase the financial burden of states and likely hurt the quality of the program as they scramble to cut costs and benefits to let the air out of bloated budgets. As the old saying in economics goes: "there is no such thing as a free lunch." The money to pay for the expansion will have to come from somewhere.

If a state like Texas is worried about new financial burdens caused by the expansion of the program, some states could save some amount of money from the changes in eligibility. Minnesota, for instance, currently permits working families to enroll in Medicaid if their income is lower than 275 percent of the federal poverty line. Under ObamaCare, the threshold will be pushed down to 133 percent. The number of working families on Medicaid in Minnesota is thus likely to drop significantly, with those who lose their eligibility given subsidies to buy health insurance on the state's new exchange.

Since the federal government pays for the entire cost of the subsidies given out to individuals who buy health insurance through the exchanges, Minnesota will save some money because of this change. Its total cost for Medicaid, however, might stay the same, or even go up, because childless adults will now be added to the program's rolls within the state, and the addition of these individuals could more than offset those who moved from Medicaid to a subsidized exchange.

REMEMBER THE "CORNHUSKER KICKBACK"?

One of the biggest controversies during the national debate over ObamaCare involved the backroom deal between Senator Ben Nelson and the Democratic leadership in the Senate. In return for his vote in favor of the healthcare reform legislation proposed by his party, Nelson's home state of Nebraska was promised special treatment which significantly lowered the amount it had to pay to cover "newly eligible" Medicaid enrollees. When news of the deal became public it triggered widespread outrage, with the loudest protests coming from Arnold Schwarzenegger, the only Republican governor to support ObamaCare. He demanded that California and every other state in the country get the same deal given to Nebraska. In the end that's what happened, defusing the anger over the "Cornhusker Kickback," but increasing the cost of ObamaCare at the federal level.

Strengthening Medicaid for the ObamaCare Expansion

ObamaCare includes a number of key provisions that will help strengthen Medicaid before and during its dramatic expansion:

- **Increased Medicaid Payment Rates** — One of the biggest problems with Medicaid over the years has been the difficulty many recipients have had finding doctors to take them on as patients. ObamaCare tries to fix this problem by increasing Medicaid payment rates for primary care doctors, including those in family, general internal, and pediatric medicine. The new rates will be raised to Medicare levels in 2014 and expire at the end of that year.

- **More Funding For Children's Insurance Health Program (CHIP)** — Under ObamaCare each state will receive a 23 percent increase in their CHIP funding up to a ceiling of 100 percent. Since the federal government already covers 65 percent or more of CHIP in most states, the program will largely be paid for in full by the federal government in 2014 and after. In addition, children who are excluded from CHIP because of enrollment limits will be able to get tax credits for insurance obtained through their state's healthcare exchange.

HEALTH INSURANCE EXCHANGES

7

I N THE LAST CHAPTER we discussed the expansion of Medicaid. Now we move on to ObamaCare's second big carrot: health insurance exchanges in every state. The collective importance of the exchanges cannot be overstated as they will function as the brain of the new healthcare system with direct links connecting them to Medicaid and the private insurance market. Over time, they will probably begin to encroach on employer-based insurance, starting with small businesses and eventually affecting businesses of all sizes.

	TAB. 7-1: MEDICAID EXPANSION — MANDATE & GOVERNMENT ASSISTANCE		
The Stick	**The Individual Mandate**		
	Every one has to get health insurance or pay fine		
	↓	↓	↓
The Carrots	**Government Assistance in the Form of ...**		
	Medicaid Expansion	Exchanges	Small Businesses
	Fully Subsidized	Partially Subsidized (on Sliding Scale)	Tax Credits (on Sliding Scale)

The future of the new healthcare law will depend very much on the exchanges. If they fail, ObamaCare will likely fail with them. If they succeed, healthcare in the United States will be transformed and a decade or more down the road the current employer-based system could be largely replaced by government-controlled, exchange-based insurance.

What Is a Health Insurance Exchange?

Simply put, a health insurance exchange is a marketplace very much like your neighborhood supermarket. When you need groceries, you visit your store to buy the products you need based on the benefits they offer you relative to their price. A health insurance exchange works the same way except the product isn't milk or cereal, but health insurance.

> **" Originally a Republican idea, the state insurance exchanges mandated under the Affordable Care Act (ACA) will offer a menu of private insurance plans to pick and choose from, all with a required set of minimum benefits, to those without employer-sponsored health insurance."**

The exchanges at the heart of ObamaCare (referred to officially in the legislation as the "American Health Benefit Exchanges") differ, however, from your neighborhood supermarket in a few important ways. For one thing, they're government regulated, meaning that the insurance sold to consumers has to meet specific quality standards. For another, some of the people who shop at the exchange will be provided money by the government to reduce the price they pay for insurance.

Each state must have an exchange because of a provision of the law which says that if any state refuses to create one for its residents by 2014 (some have already threatened non-compliance) the federal government will create and manage it for them. Given the loud opposition from many states, fueled mostly by their dissatisfaction with the expansion of Medicaid, federally run exchanges are likely in some states.

As of mid-2012 only 16 of the nation's 50 states had begun to create their ObamaCare health exchange. Most of the rest are considering it. But four states have already announced they will not create an exchange, including Alaska. Governor Sean Parnell said that "allocating state dollars and personnel to design and implement an exchange is the most expensive option." In other words, he wants Washington to pick up the full cost for its creation and operation.

Will Exchanges Improve the Healthcare System?

If you didn't hear much about the health insurance exchanges in the debate over ObamaCare, there's a reason. Compared to other parts of the new law, they are free of controversy. Conservatives like that they are competitive marketplaces while liberals like the way they protect consumers and subsidize their purchases. Enjoying support from many on both sides of the political fence, the exchanges are expected to improve the current system in a number of ways:

- **Increased Choice** — Just as multiple brands of cereal can be found in an aisle of the supermarket, multiple health insurance plans will be housed in each exchange where consumers will be able to easily compare plans to one another based on their price and quality.

- **Standardization** — Plans sold through the exchange by different insurance companies must contain identical levels of benefits at specific tiers of coverage so consumers can make "apples-to-apples" comparisons between the plans.

- **Consumer Protection** — Consumers will have confidence that they are not being sold an inferior policy because each plan must cover "essential health benefits" (See Appendix A).

- **Economies of Scale** — Because the exchanges will be places where hundreds of thousands (and in some cases millions) of consumers shop, they will foster healthy competition among insurance companies. As a consequence, prices should come down as quality goes up.

As vocal as Republicans have been in criticizing ObamaCare, former U.S. Senator Bill Frist, a heart transplant surgeon and party elder who once served as Majority Leader of the U.S. Senate, is not a knee-jerk opponent of the new law. He is a big supporter of the exchanges and wrote an editorial in their favor, saying: "Originally a Republican idea, the state insurance exchanges mandated under the Affordable Care Act (ACA) will offer a menu of private insurance plans to pick and choose from, all with a required set of minimum benefits, to those without employer-sponsored health insurance."

"State exchanges are the solution," wrote Frist. "They represent the federalist ideal of states as 'laboratories for democracy.' We are seeing 50 states each designing a model that is right for them, empowered to take into account their individual cultures, politics, economies and demographics. While much planning has yet to be done, we are already seeing a huge range in state models. I love the diversity and the innovation."

Frist may be right to be enthusiastic about the exchanges. Right now, insurers spend an estimated $25 billion a year on marketing and distribution of their insurance policies — a significant amount of which can be saved by automating the process with an Internet portal.

Americans are accustomed to buying all types of products over the Internet, from cars to books to airplane tickets. Health insurance, however, has been a laggard in this regard. According to Price Waterhouse, only about 5 percent of health insurance policies are currently bought online. When the ObamaCare health exchanges begin to operate, this number will rise dramatically, empowering buyers and sellers of insurance alike.

You'll be able to shop for health insurance in your state's exchange by visiting the government office that manages it. If you prefer, you can buy an insurance plan over the phone (via a toll-free number) or through the exchange's website (most sales will flow through this convenient portal). The goal is to make the whole shopping and buying process as easy as possible for the consumer. As Peter Lee, the head of the new California health exchange put it, buying health insurance should now become "as easy as buying a book on Amazon."

If it suits a state's needs, it may create multiple exchanges within its borders as long as each one serves a distinct geographic area within the state. Heavily populated states like California, for instance, could create one exchange to serve the northern part of its geography and another to serve the southern part.

On the other end of the spectrum, less populated states will be able to form a regional health insurance exchange with neighboring states, so that Hawaii, Alaska, Washington and Oregon could, if they choose, form a single "Pacific Exchange" to increase risk pools and better serve their residents.

What About a Single National Exchange?

You might be wondering: Why not just create a single health insurance exchange that would serve the entire country?

Such an exchange would make it possible to buy health insurance across state lines, something which is not legally permitted today. Critics of ObamaCare strongly support interstate commerce of this kind. They argue that one of the ways to bring down healthcare costs is to make health insurance more competitive by allowing a person in New Jersey, for instance, to buy a policy from an insurance company in Nevada.

A national exchange would seem to be both intrinsically feasible and politically viable. Appearances can be deceiving, however. If we go back to the presidential campaign of 2008, then-candidate Barack Obama actually promised to create a single national health insurance exchange. But once he entered office, the widespread fears that his reform package represented a government takeover of the healthcare system pushed him away from that idea. In the end, a national exchange became untenable.

That may not have been a bad outcome for the country. After all, the functional knowledge needed to regulate health insurance currently resides at the state level (each has its own rules and mandates governing the sale of health insurance). It's probably sensible to leverage this expertise where it exists rather than try to reinvent the wheel by replacing it with a new federal bureaucracy that would have no experience doing the same tasks. A single national exchange can always be created at a later date if needed.

Massachusetts' Health Connector

For a real world example of what a health insurance exchange looks like, visit the Massachusetts' Health Connector website at *www. mahealthconnector.org*. The state's healthcare system — sometimes referred to as "RomneyCare" for former Governor Mitt Romney, who signed the law that created it in 2006 — is a working prototype for the ObamaCare exchanges that all Americans will see in their states in 2014.

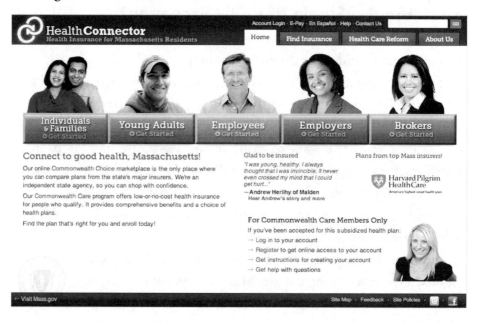

In the Massachusetts exchange the state government acts as the buyer of health insurance from five approved insurance providers. It negotiates prices and benefits for various tiers of coverage to help get the best deal for its residents, and only those plans that receive its stamp of approval are made available for purchase. The ObamaCare exchanges will work in much the same way, although each state will enjoy a certain amount of flexibility in determining its own management approach.

Besides Massachusetts there is only one other health insurance exchange operating in the United States right now — a much smaller one in Utah that sells insurance to small businesses. The Utah exchange is more open than the Connector in Massachusetts, allowing a wide range of insurance companies to sell policies directly to buyers and letting free market forces set prices.

The exchanges created by ObamaCare that begin operating in 2014 will be able to choose either of these management philosophies or something in between. In California, former Governor Arnold Schwarzenegger set in motion the process of creating that state's exchange in 2010. Much to the delight of President Obama, he did so using the Massachusetts model as a template, making it clear that the state government in Sacramento would be a vigilant gatekeeper and manager of its exchange with tight controls.

OBAMACARE'S TEMPLATE — THE MASSACHUSETTS EXAMPLE

Like ObamaCare, the Massachusetts healthcare system is powered by an individual mandate which compels participation in the system through the threat of a financial penalty and is built around a heavily subsidized exchange where regulated insurance plans can be bought at affordable prices.

The question naturally arises: How has the Massachusetts system worked since its creation? The answer will give us some indication about how ObamaCare would perform if it was fully implemented.

According to an in-depth study by the conservative Beacon Hill Institute, "RomneyCare" has hurt the state significantly by:

- Costing it almost 20,000 jobs
- Driving up health insurance costs by more than $4 billion
- Lowering disposable income per household by almost $400

On the positive side, Massachusetts now has the highest level of healthcare coverage in the country, with only about 3 percent of its population uninsured. Most of the newly insured have received coverage through subsidies and about half pay nothing at all for their insurance, leaving state taxpayers to pick up the bill. ObamaCare is likely to do much the same on a national scale.

Despite RomneyCare's promises to bring down healthcare costs (they were eerily similar to ObamaCare's promises back in 2008), the typical family of four in Massachusetts now pays the highest health insurance premiums in the country, according to the Commonwealth Fund, a non-profit healthcare foundation.

If there is a lesson to be learned from the Massachusetts example it appears to be that it will be very costly to implement a similar system across the entire United States as it will likely lead to more expensive health insurance, fewer jobs and a greater financial burden for taxpayers.

The number of uninsured Americans will fall dramatically, but the price for this expansion of healthcare coverage will put another blot on the nation's already ugly balance sheet. The Massachusetts healthcare system is, in short, a case study that makes a persuasive argument that ObamaCare may, on the whole, reduce the number of uninsured residents, but at a significant cost to American taxpayers and insurance policyholders.

Are Exchanges Really Necessary?

In striving to decrease the uninsured population, ObamaCare dramatically expands Medicaid and in the process gives health insurance to 15 million people at no direct cost to them (this figure assumes all states participate in the expansion of the program). But as bold and sweeping as that action is, it still would leave more than 20 million Americans without health insurance in 2019.

The authors of ObamaCare turned to health insurance exchanges as the means to expand coverage to this portion of the uninsured population because they saw that the exchange in Massachusetts had helped that state secure health insurance for 97 percent of its residents.

Taking something that has worked within one state and spreading it to other states is not a new idea (back in the 1930s Supreme Court Justice Louis Brandeis famously called the states the great "laboratories of democracy"), but rarely has a program of such importance been expanded to the entire country in the way the ObamaCare exchanges promise to do.

By 2019 roughly 25 million people are expected to use the exchanges to obtain quality coverage at an affordable cost. This includes 16 million people who would otherwise be uninsured plus an additional 9 million Americans from the private and employer-based insurance markets who will be attracted by the low cost and high value of exchange insurance plans.

Eligibility to Use the Exchanges

Who exactly will be eligible to buy health insurance on the exchanges? Pretty much every American will be allowed into the exchange in their state when they want to buy insurance for themselves, but there are some additional rules governing eligibility.

- **Illegal Aliens Excluded** — Only U.S. citizens and legal immigrants who are not incarcerated will be able to use the exchanges. Legal immigrants are not eligible for Medicaid benefits during their first five years in the United States, but those who would have qualified for the program if they were here long enough will be able to receive government financial assistance if they want to buy insurance through the exchange while they wait to get into Medicaid.

- **Employees Who Have Poor Coverage** — The exchanges were created mostly with the private health insurance market in mind, to help reduce the cost for single individuals and families trying to buy coverage on their own. The exchanges, however, are also open to workers whose employers offer them health insurance that does not cover at least 60 percent of their medical costs or if the employee's share of premiums exceeds 9.5 percent of their wages.

- **Small Businesses** — Companies with up to 100 employees may buy health insurance for their employees through an exchange (the exchange for businesses — called the "Small Business Health Options Program" or SHOP — will be kept separate from those for individuals in each state). Beginning in 2017 states will be allowed, if they choose, to let companies with more than 100 employees buy insurance through the exchanges.

There's a good reason to keep big businesses out of the exchanges during the initial phase-in period. They tend to have a relatively large share of older, less healthy employees enrolled in their insurance plans. If members of this higher risk group were permitted to immediately enter the exchanges, they could push the price of premiums upward by their presence and squeeze out smaller businesses trying to buy affordable insurance.

Will large businesses use the exchanges if they are eventually allowed into them? The answer will depend on how well the exchanges function between 2014 and 2017. If they create a marketplace where prices are low, companies of all sizes will be attracted to them, especially if they can also escape the administrative burden of managing healthcare for their employees by buying insurance from an exchange.

Four Standardized Plans:
Bronze, Silver, Gold, and Platinum

Buying a health insurance plan that meets all your needs is not an easy task. For one thing, it's often hard to know the value of what you're buying. With so many different parts of insurance coverage and so much fine print (much of it written in hard-to-understand legalese), it's not uncommon to discover that your insurance doesn't cover a condition that you thought it did. And this discovery usually happens right when you need the coverage in question.

One of the biggest benefits of the exchanges is that they will cut through this complexity and simplify the decision-making process for those who go to buy health insurance. Each state's exchange will be required to offer four standardized insurance plans which collectively will provide a range of coverage, low to high. These plans will be designated "Bronze," "Silver," "Gold," and "Platinum," with each providing a successively higher amount of coverage.

The quality of these plans should also be high as each one, regardless of the amount of coverage it offers, will be required to include so-called "essential health benefits." All health insurance plans sold outside the exchanges in the individual and small group market will be required to do the same, raising the quality of health insurance everywhere in the United States.

What exactly are "essential health benefits"? In November 2012, the Department of Health and Human Services released a list of the broad areas that will be part of the essential health benefits. By the time the exchanges open in 2014 HHS will have established more details of the health benefits list that will comprise a baseline level of coverage that all plans sold on and off an exchange must have. Generally speaking, these benefits will be comparable to what can be found in a typical employer-based plan today.

After this minimum level of benefits is met, the tiers of insurance coverage will differ based on their "actuarial value." This is the amount of financial coverage that the plan offers, on average, to its participants. The Bronze plan will offer the lowest amount of coverage, with 60 percent of medical costs covered on average, followed by the Silver plan at 70 percent, the Gold plan at 80 percent, and the Platinum plan at 90 percent. The price of plan premiums will follow this escalating hierarchy with the Silver plan costing more than the Bronze plan and so forth.

TAB. 7-2: **PAYING FOR NEW MEDICAID ENROLLEES UNDER OBAMACARE***				
Plan Name	**Out-of-Pocket Limits*** Individuals	Families	**Covers "Essential Health Benefits"***	**Percent of Costs Covered by Plan**
Bronze	$5,950	$11,900	Yes	60%
Silver	$5,950	$11,900	Yes	70%
Gold	$5,950	$11,900	Yes	80%
Platinum	$5,950	$11,900	Yes	90%

*Pegged to Health Savings Account levels in 2010 and assumes income above 400% of federal poverty level. Out-of-pocket limits decrease for lower income levels.
**Not yet defined by the Department of Health & Human Services

Those who receive government subsidies to buy insurance through an exchange will benefit by gaining access to plans with actuarial values they would not otherwise be able to afford. In addition, the baseline out-of-pocket limit for each plan will match the limits that apply to Health Savings Accounts ($5,950 for individuals and $11,900 for families in 2010). Those who receive government subsidies will see their out-of-pocket limits lowered from these levels as a consequence of the financial assistance they receive just as their premiums will be lowered.

A "Catastrophic" Insurance Plan for Those Under Age 30

If you're under the age of 30 and don't feel the need to buy health insurance but are compelled to do so because of the individual mandate, a special "catastrophic" insurance plan will be available to you and to those who are exempt from the mandate. The plan will be less expensive than the Bronze plan (i.e., it will cover less than 60 percent of the medical costs on average) and will include prevention benefits and three annual visits to your primary care doctor. In addition, young adults up to the age of 26 who are looking to get around the individual mandate will be allowed under ObamaCare to remain a dependent covered by their parents' insurance.

An Optional "Basic Health Plan" for Each State

Although ObamaCare requires each state to set up an exchange, it also gives states flexibility in managing its size. Under the new law, each state can create a so-called "Basic Health Plan" for uninsured individuals with incomes between 133 percent and 200 percent of the federal poverty line ($14,440 to $21,660 in 2010).

This Basic Health Plan must include the "essential health benefits" offered by the Bronze, Silver, Gold, and Platinum plans through the exchange and must ensure that its enrollees do not pay more than they would have if they purchased them independently.

States offering a Basic Health Plan will receive 95 percent of the money that would have been paid by the federal government in subsidies to those individuals covered by it. Because government funds will be redirected in this way, individuals who enroll in such plans will not be able to get subsidies through the exchange.

Standards for Insurance Sellers

In addition to establishing different tiers of health insurance offered through each exchange, the government will measure and rate the quality of the insurance plans and the companies that sell them based on key performance metrics such as enrollment levels, the number of people dropping out of a plan and the amount of denied claims.

In order to sell plans through an exchange, insurance companies will be required to meet certain standards. For instance, they will need to market their plans according to government regulations, support their plans with adequate provider networks, make enrollment easy, and provide assistance to consumers. If they don't do these things, insurers could receive a low performance rating, which would warn consumers of the danger of doing business with them. In a worst-case scenario, they could be prohibited from selling through an exchange altogether.

The government's power to single out and banish an insurance company from the exchanges is perhaps its most powerful regulatory weapon. If this weapon is used (it probably won't be in most cases), it could very well put an insurer out of business.

A Range of Exchange Subsidies

Financial assistance from the federal government will be offered through the exchanges to all Americans who qualify. It will come in two forms, both of which will lower the price of the health insurance plan that a consumer wishes to buy:

- Lower Premiums

- Lower Out-of-Pocket Limits

Lower Premiums

Subsidies will be provided based on where a person's income level falls on a sliding scale. Those whose income falls in the bottom of the scale (the floor is 133 percent of the federal poverty line) will receive the most government assistance and those whose income reaches the top of the scale (the ceiling is 400 percent of the poverty line) will receive the least. Those whose income exceeds the ceiling level will not receive subsidies.

In 2010 dollars that means a family of four will qualify for a subsidy when they buy through an exchange if their income falls between $29,328 and $88,200, with the amount of the subsidy depending on their income level within this range.

A family of four on the high end of the scale will pay a maximum of 9.5 percent of their $88,200 annual income — or $8,379 per year for their health insurance premium. On the bottom end of the scale, a family of four with an income of $29,327 will only have to pay 2 percent of their income — or $587 per year for the same plan that cost the higher income family $8,379.

TAB. 7-3: **COST OF PREMIUMS ON HEALTH EXCHANGES FOR FAMILY OF FOUR**				
Percent of Federal Poverty Level	**Income Level***	**Percent of Income**	**Maximum Annual Premium**	**Premium Per Month**
400%	$88,200	9.5%	$8,379	$698
300%	$66,150	9.5%	$6,284	$524
250%	$55,125	8.1%	$4,438	$370
200%	$44,100	6.3%	$2,778	$232
150%	$33,075	4.0%	$1,323	$110
133%	$29,327	2.0%	$587	$49

*For a family of four in 2010 the federal poverty level is $22,050.

Lower Out-of-Pocket Limits

Government assistance on the exchanges is also provided in the form of lower out-of-pocket limits, which are the levels that an individual or family must pay before their insurance plan begins to cover their medical expenses.

Once again, the subsidies are given out according to a sliding scale pegged to the federal poverty line, with people in the lowest income range receiving the most help. The baseline out-of-pocket limit on each exchange is equal to the out-of-pocket limit for Health Savings Accounts (currently $5,950 for individuals and $11,900 for families) and is lowered from that ceiling level according to where an income level falls in the range.

? DID YOU KNOW . . .
Insurance plans sold through a state exchange may cover abortions, but government money may be used only in cases involving rape, incest or danger to the mother's life.

TAB. 7-4: OUT-OF-POCKET LIMITS BASED ON FEDERAL POVERTY LEVEL			
Percent of Federal Poverty Level	**Individual**	**Percent of Health Savings Account**	**Families**
Above 400% (Health Saving Account Level)	$5,950	100%	$11,900
300 to 400%	$3,987	67%	$7,933
200 to 299%	$2,975	50%	$5,950
100 to 199%	$1,983	33%	$3,967

In 2010 dollars this means that a family with an income that falls in the lowest range (100 to 199 percent of the federal poverty level) will reach its out-of-pocket limit at $3,967 — or 33 percent of the amount for a Health Savings Account ($11,900) used by a high-income family.

Increased "Actuarial Value" of Plans

The end result of lower premiums and out-of-pocket limits because of government subsidies will mean an increased "actuarial value" (the percentage of medical costs covered on average for each beneficiary) for the plans sold to low-income Americans through an exchange.

Pegged to the Silver Plan on the exchange at 400 percent of the federal poverty level, the subsidies increase the actuarial value of the plan as the income level drops. For example, at the 400 percent income level ($88,200) the Silver Plan covers 70 percent of medical costs on average, while at the bottom end of the income range (133 percent of the federal poverty level) it covers 94 percent of medical costs.

TAB. 7-5: **OUT-OF-POCKET LIMITS BASED ON FEDERAL POVERTY LEVEL**			
Percent of Federal Poverty Level	Income Level*	Out-Of Pocket Limit	% Of Medical Cost Plan Covers
400%	$88,200	$7,933	70%
300%	$66,150	$5,950	70%
250%	$55,125	$5,950	73%
200%	$44,100	$3,967	87%
150%	$33,075	$3,967	94%
133%	$29,327	$3,967	94%

*Family of four

Keep in mind that the "actuarial value" is an average amount of coverage for all the participants in a particular plan. Depending on the total amount of medical costs, a plan will cover a higher percentage of costs for some plan members than for others. For instance, someone who has $100,000 in medical costs will obviously have more of their expenses paid for by their insurance than someone who has expenses below their out-of-pocket limit.

WHAT ABOUT ABORTION AND CONTRACEPTION COVERAGE?

Insurance plans sold through an exchange may cover abortions, but government money may be used only in cases involving rape, incest or danger to the mother's life. The Hyde Amendment passed in the 1980s forbids the use of taxpayer funds to subsidize abortions, with the exceptions noted, and ObamaCare conforms to this law. Therefore, if someone buys a subsidized insurance plan through an exchange with abortion coverage, they will have to make two separate payments, one of which may be subsidized by the government and one (which covers the abortion) which may not.

Contraception is not as controversial as abortion, but it's an important issue for some, notably conservative Catholics. Those who have moral qualms about contraception have protested the Obama administration's decision to force all insurers to provide contraception to women without a co-pay. At the time this book went to print, 23 lawsuits had been filed in federal court arguing that this mandate violated the religious freedom guaranteed by the Constitution.

We are a long way off from a final resolution of the matter, but in an attempt to lessen the controversy the White House has agreed to selectively issue waivers in the short term which permit religiously affiliated organizations with moral objections to sidestep the new regulation for the time being. Private employers, however, are not exempt.

What will the Supreme Court decide? As seen by the surprise of so many experts when the court upheld the individual mandate as constitutional, predicting its decisions is far from easy. Justice Ruth Bader Ginsburg, a staunch liberal who voted to uphold the individual mandate, nonetheless did so in such a way that suggests that she does not like the contraception mandate as much.

Her observation suggests that she may vote to strike down the contraception mandate, which does not bode well for its future as she would likely be joined by the four justices who voted to strike down the individual mandate. In what appeared to be a warning shot across the bow of the Obama White House, Ginsburg wrote: "A mandate to purchase a particular product would be unconstitutional if, for example, the edict impermissibly abridged the freedom of speech, interfered with the free exercise of religion or infringed on a liberty interest protected by the Due Process Clause."

Affordable Care Act (P.L. 111-148)

What Happened to the "Public Option"?

During the national debate over ObamaCare many Americans came to believe that the United States government was trying to take over healthcare in the country through a "public option" that would create a so-called "single-payer" system similar to what Canada uses today. This was the never the case.

In reality, the "public option" was merely a government-run insurance plan meant as an alternative to the plans sold by private insurance companies on the exchanges. All insurance sellers under this scheme, including the government, would have sold the same Bronze, Silver, Gold, and Platinum plans as everyone else.

Nonetheless, critics of the "public option" worried that the government's plan would overwhelm private insurance plans and destroy the competitive aspect of the exchanges. This was a reasonable fear. With its immense size and resources, the federal government could charge the lowest prices with the stroke of a bureaucrat's pen. Lower prices produced in this way would have proven attractive to consumers in the short term, but they would have opened up a door that many feared would lead directly to socialized medicine in the United States.

Still, despite what the critics said about the "public option," its impact would have been limited in the short term to the exchanges and those are expected to be used by less than 10 percent of the American population by 2019. In this sense, there was little chance of ObamaCare completely taking over healthcare in the country. Even if the government insurance plan had marginalized private insurance plans sold on the exchanges, it still would have left at least 90 percent of Americans getting their health insurance from a source other than the "public option" insurance plan that could be found only through an exchange.

In the end the critics won the argument when Senator Joe Lieberman of Connecticut refused to vote for Obama's plan with a "public option." Congress then stripped the public option out of the final legislation, gaining Lieberman's crucial vote for passage.

INCENTIVES FOR SMALL BUSINESSES

8

THE THIRD BIG CARROT of ObamaCare helps decrease the number of uninsured by offering tax credits to some small businesses that provide coverage for their employees.

TAB. 8-1: **MEDICAID EXPANSION —** **MANDATE & GOVERNMENT ASSISTANCE**			
	The Individual Mandate		
The Stick	**Every one has to get health insurance or pay fine**		
	↓	↓	↓
	Government Assistance in the Form of . . .		
The Carrots	**Medicaid Expansion**	**Exchanges**	**Small Businesses**
	Fully Subsidized	**Partially Subsidized** (on Sliding Scale)	**Tax Credits** (on Sliding Scale)

Rapidly rising healthcare costs hurt most Americans, but small businesses are particularly vulnerable because these firms have to pay more per employee for health insurance than larger businesses.

On average, premiums are about 20 percent higher for small businesses compared to large businesses, with their plan enrollees having to pay higher deductibles. Administrative costs are even higher and, according to one study, are about four times more than those of a typical big business on a per worker basis. Because of this large financial burden, many small businesses eliminate jobs or don't hire new workers.

❓ DID YOU KNOW . . .

The small business tax credit is designed to preserve the current employer-based healthcare system, at least in the short term (it expires at the end of 2015).

The divide between large businesses and small ones is a wide gulf. In Texas, for example, a robust 95 percent of businesses with 50 or more workers provide health insurance to their employees, while only 31 percent of those with less than 50 workers do the same. Looking under the surface of these numbers, they suggest not only a larger financial burden for smaller businesses, but also that they do not need to attract workers with health insurance the way large businesses do, which operate in a much more competitive labor market.

Seen in this light, ObamaCare is good news for those who work for small businesses. These individuals, many of whom do not have health insurance or are forced to buy it at an expensive price on the private market, will now be able to use the exchanges in their states to obtain it for an affordable amount. In many cases they will be eligible for a government-provided subsidy to defray the costs of their purchases, making the plan even more financially attractive.

With an exchange-based insurance plan, workers will also enjoy more freedom to switch jobs or work on their own. Because workers in this situation will no longer be anchored to their employers to get coverage, increasing numbers of them may become freelancers. These positive developments, however, could come with a negative effect, too.

That's because when the new exchanges begin to operate in 2014 there will be even less incentive for small businesses to offer their employees health insurance, especially those who are paid very low wages. More low-wage workers will therefore turn to state exchanges to get health insurance than might otherwise be the case.

In Texas, many small businesses that currently provide coverage to their workers may drop such benefits after 2014. According to a survey conducted by Mercer, a benefits consulting firm, about 20 percent of small businesses are expected to drop their coverage once the exchanges begin to operate. If this happens, it will escalate a trend already underway. About 20 percent fewer small businesses today provide coverage for their workers than a decade ago (compared to a 99 percent health insurance retention rate among large businesses).

To prevent this snowball effect, ObamaCare provides a tax credit to encourage small businesses to offer health insurance to their workers, both now and after the exchanges open (the tax credit is intentionally increased in 2014 for this reason).

The small business tax credit is designed to preserve the current employer-based healthcare system, at least in the short term (it expires at the end of 2015). But, the tax credit is more of a firewall put in place to prevent small businesses from completely eliminating their health insurance plans.

It's an open question whether or not the tax credit will be enough to save employer-based health insurance provided by small businesses in the long run. If the exchanges prove successful, pressure will likely build on these businesses to drop coverage for their workers, even with a big tax credit providing an incentive to do the opposite. If the tax credit is not renewed when it expires at the end of 2015, that pressure will only increase.

> **❓ DID YOU KNOW . . .**
>
> **Right now, a company that has up to 10 employees, average annual wages under $25,000 and contributes to at least 50% of their healthcare premium costs is eligible for a 35% tax credit against the amount it pays for its workers' insurance.**

According to a report by Bernstein Research, since the small business tax credit went into effect in 2010 it has had a positive effect as businesses with fewer than 10 employees that offered health insurance to their workers jumped from 46 to 59 percent that first year alone.

SHOP Health Insurance Exchanges

ObamaCare's help for small businesses goes beyond tax credits. No longer will a small business have to buy insurance from a weak, isolated position as a single entity with only a handful of employees. Buying through new business healthcare exchanges will allow them to become part of a much larger risk pool – eliminating one of the big reasons small firms have historically paid more for health insurance than larger companies.

Administered by a governmental agency or non-profit organization, the SHOP exchanges (officially called the "Small Business Health Options Program") will at first only be open to businesses with up to 100 employees. Starting in 2017 states will be permitted, if they choose, to open up their exchanges to businesses with more than 100 employees. If before that time a small business that has bought insurance through SHOP grows in excess of 100 employees, it will be able to remain in the exchange regardless of how big it becomes.

The long-term success of ObamaCare will depend on how much the exchanges attract the nation's business community. If the attraction is strong, we could see large companies begin to buy health insurance for their employees through SHOP instead of directly from insurance companies themselves. That movement could, in turn, undermine the employer-based insurance system that now dominates the nation's healthcare landscape, if not replace it altogether.

Tax Credits to Use SHOP Exchanges

The simplified purchasing process and the lower prices expected to come with the SHOP exchanges should attract small businesses, but ObamaCare provides an additional incentive in the form of a tax credit. Businesses with up to 25 employees will be eligible for a tax credit of a specific amount based on the number of employees they have, the average annual wages their employees earn and the business's share of the premium cost.

TAB. 8-2: **TAX CREDITS FOR SMALL BUSINESSES**				
	For Small Businesses With:			
Dates Effective	**Number of Employees**	**Average Annual Wages**	**Contribution to Premium Cost**	**Tax Credit**
2010 to 2013	1 to 10	Under $25,000	50% or more	35%
	11 to 25			< 35%
	Over 25			None
2014 to 2015	1 to 10	Under $25,000	50% or more	50%
	11 to 25			< 50%
	Over 25			None

Right now, a company that has up to 10 employees, average annual wages under $25,000 and contributes to at least 50 percent of their healthcare premium costs is eligible for a 35 percent tax credit against the amount it pays for its workers' insurance.

Under the same conditions, a small business with 11 to 25 employees will receive lower credits based on a sliding scale until the credit disappears with 26 or more employees. Beginning in 2014, the tax credit will rise to a maximum of 50 percent for two years before it expires, assuming Congress does not decide to extend it into 2016 and beyond.

Tax-exempt small businesses that meet these conditions will be able to receive a tax credit of 25 percent against the amount they pay to insure their workers from 2010 to 2013. The credit will rise to 35 percent in 2014 and expire at the end of 2015.

> **? DID YOU KNOW . . .**
> Big businesses that don't offer workers health insurance will pay fines of $2,000 for every full-time employee who receives a government subsidy for purchasing coverage through an exchange, excluding the first 30 employees.

Small Businesses Exempt From Penalties

Understanding that small businesses are less able to bear financial burdens than bigger businesses, the authors of ObamaCare exempt them from penalties it imposes on companies with more than 50 employees that don't provide health coverage. Large businesses will risk financial fines if they:

- Do not offer their employees health insurance

- Offer health insurance that is low quality

In either situation, employees who are compelled by the individual mandate to obtain health insurance could turn away from their employer and buy coverage on their state's exchange. The minute they do and receive a government subsidy when buying their insurance plan, the company they work for (assuming it has more than 50 employees) will incur financial penalties. In case you were wondering, the new law prevents employers from retaliating against an employee who triggers these corporate penalties by their decision to buy subsidized insurance through an exchange.

TAB. 8-3: PENALTY FOR EMPLOYERS WITH 50+ EMPLOYEES WHO HAVE AN EMPLOYEE WHO GETS GOVERNMENT FINANCIAL ASSISTANCE ON A HEALTH EXCHANGE		
Type of Employer:	Employer Does Not Offer Coverage	Employer Does Offer Coverage
		The lesser of...
Penalty Per Full-Time Employee	$2,000	$2,000
		Or
Penalty Per Employee Who Gets Tax Credit on Exchange	NA	$3,000
Penalty Applies To:	Only for Employees #31 and over	All Employees

Businesses that don't offer workers health insurance will pay fines of $2,000 for every full-time employee who receives a government subsidy for purchasing coverage through an exchange, excluding the first 30 employees.

If the employer does offer coverage and an employee nonetheless receives a government subsidy when buying through an exchange (suggesting that the employer's coverage is either too expensive or of poor quality), the employer will also have to pay a fine. That amount will be the lesser of two sums: either $2,000 per full-time employee or $3,000 for each employee who receives a subsidy on the exchange.

The 50-worker threshold could become an important line of demarcation for some small businesses because once they cross it they become subject to the $2,000 fine per worker if they don't provide health insurance. The issue has raised some questions about what constitutes a worker under the new law. The Health and Human Services administration will make the ultimate decision and small businesses are lobbying to ensure that they are not penalized for hiring part-time and seasonal workers.

Another bone of contention: An entrepreneur who owns a number of small businesses is right now considered one business conglomerate by the government, when determining the 50-worker threshold.

Some Workers Will Lose Their Employer-Based Plans

ObamaCare will have a significant impact on businesses in the United States, forcing them to make new calculations and decisions about whether or not they should provide health insurance to their workers.

Over the last decade small businesses have increasingly dropped coverage as financial burdens from rising healthcare costs have become unbearable. This trend will likely increase when the new state health exchanges begin to operate in 2014, bringing with them a government-subsidized alternative that will entice many workers to use them, letting small businesses off the hook.

? DID YOU KNOW . . .
ObamaCare is, on the whole, great news for those who work for small business. If your company decides to pass on the tax credit and drop coverage, you can still get your insurance through a government-subsidized exchange at an affordable price. If you work for a big business, you will probably end up keeping your current employer-based plan.

In the short term, small businesses will have to determine whether or not it's in their interest to provide health insurance for their workers and receive a generous tax credit (which decreases the cost of the premiums they pay by as much as 50 percent) or to drop coverage. If they make the latter decision, the pain will be softened considerably because the state-based, government-subsidized exchanges will be available for the workers to obtain coverage at an affordable cost.

It is difficult to know what will happen, but it seems likely the trend toward fewer small businesses providing health coverage for their workers will continue, despite the tax credit offered by the government. The decision for many small businesses will boil down to whether or not they need to offer health insurance to entice new hires and keep the workers they have on the payroll.

The financial calculation that large businesses have to make will be different. They will not be able to use the exchanges and they get no tax credit from the IRS. More importantly, health insurance is, in most cases, an incentive for attracting and retaining their workers who might otherwise go to work for other companies that offer such benefits. Big businesses aren't likely to abruptly start dropping their health insurance plans in such a highly competitive labor market.

Some big businesses, however, do not compete for labor on health insurance benefits, and these will feel significant pressure to drop their coverage. Companies like McDonald's, whose labor force is large but not well paid, is in this situation. It doesn't need to provide health insurance for its workers to retain them and has already threatened to drop coverage as its health insurance costs have risen significantly due to new ObamaCare mandates, which outlaw the bare-bones "Mini-Med" plans that McDonald's currently provides to its workers.

Fearing the negative consequences that could result from health coverage elimination by McDonald's and other large companies, the White House issued waivers permitting them to sidestep the law until

2014. It remains to be seen whether or not these waivers will be extended, but they might have to be.

Large businesses will decide whether to keep providing health insurance for their workers based on the extent to which they compete with other companies for top talent. The financial penalty they will incur if they don't offer coverage will be another important consideration.

Every large business will have to pay a $2,000 fine for each worker it does not cover. With the cost of premiums per worker much higher than this amount, some companies will opt to pay the fine and drop coverage altogether.

WHAT DOES ALL THIS MEAN FOR YOU?

ObamaCare is, on the whole, great news for those who work for small businesses as defined by the legislation. If your company decides to pass on the tax credit and drop coverage, you can still get your insurance through a government-subsidized exchange at an affordable price. In this case, you would not be anchored to one company, and would have more freedom to switch jobs or work as a freelancer.

If you work for a big business, you will probably end up keeping your current employer-based plan, especially if you work for a company that competes aggressively in the labor market for workers. If you work for a company like McDonald's, which pays workers near minimum wages, you may be in greater danger. Waivers are currently preventing you from losing your coverage, but it is uncertain whether they will continue in place beyond 2014.

The 1099 Reporting Requirement Repealed

One of ObamaCare's less-noticed provisions required businesses of all sizes to account for each purchase they made in excess of $600 by sending a 1099 form documenting the purchase to the Internal Revenue Service and to the person or business who was party to the transaction.

Although the new rule would have helped the government keep track of what it's owed, it also would have created an accounting nightmare for businesses and increased their overhead costs. Small businesses, in particular, were outraged at the new requirement because their administrative capabilities are less developed than those of large businesses.

Fortunately for them, the 1099 reporting requirement was officially repealed in April 2011 with President Obama backing the effort. He had little choice as many Congressional Democrats worked aggressively for the repeal of the provision, including Senate Democrat Max Baucus, Chairman of the Senate Finance Committee, who declared: "Small businesses are the backbone of our economy in my home state of Montana and across the country, and they need to focus their efforts on creating good-paying jobs — not filing paperwork."

Employee Vouchers to Buy Through an Exchange

Businesses will also be required under a new ObamaCare rule to provide their employees with a voucher to purchase health insurance if an employee:

- Buys a health insurance plan through an exchange

- Earns less than 400 percent of the federal poverty level ($22,050 for a family of four in 2010)

- Pays a share of the employer's insurance premium that exceeds 8 percent but is less than 9.8 percent of the employee's wages

The voucher can only be used to buy insurance through the exchange. Its value must be equal to the amount that the employer would have paid if the employee were covered under the company's health insurance plan. Employers who give their workers vouchers will be free from any penalties which might otherwise occur from these workers receiving exchange subsidies.

Large Businesses Must Use Automatic Enrollment

A small, easily overlooked ObamaCare requirement will help get healthcare coverage for working Americans in a stealthy way. It compels all employers with more than 200 employees to automatically enroll their workers in company insurance plans whether the employees realize they are being enrolled or not.

Employees may leave their employer's plan, if they so choose, and in doing so can avoid paying their share of insurance premiums, but they will have to make a conscious decision to do so. Most people, of course, choose to enroll in their employer's insurance plan out of convenience or because they realize that their employer pays most of the cost. In this sense, the automatic enrollment provision of ObamaCare is not a big deal and will insulate workers from the individual mandate's financial penalty, but it highlights the law's underlying paternalistic approach.

PART III
COSTS WILL BEND UP, NOT DOWN

"Most of us agree [ObamaCare] will probably boost the insured population and you could probably give it an A. But I think it gets an F on bending the cost curve up instead of down."
— Charles Boorady, a managing director with Credit Suisse

MORE BENEFITS, HIGHER COSTS

EVERY AMERICAN, WHETHER A SUPPORTER of ObamaCare or not, should find the goals of the healthcare reform package President Obama signed into law in March 2010 commendable. We should all want as many Americans as possible to have health insurance because virtually everyone will one day need it. And we should all want Americans to be able to obtain quality healthcare at reasonable prices.

The controversy that continues to swirl around ObamaCare is not about its goals, but rather is about how we achieve the ends most of us want. The core debate is really about the price of reform, with some Americans naturally willing to pay more for improvements to a functioning, albeit flawed, system than others.

Given the emphasis that the new law puts behind decreasing the uninsured population, and the massive amount of money that will be spent to achieve that end by expanding Medicaid and providing subsidized health insurance through exchanges, it's probable that this — the number one goal of ObamaCare — will be achieved.

? DID YOU KNOW . . .

There are more than three times as many Magnetic Resonance Imaging (MRI) devices in the United States per capita as in any other developed nation.

Spending $899 billion toward this end while cutting Medicare pretty much guarantees its success. Whether or not it's worth that stratospheric price is an altogether different question that continues to divide the American people nearly three years after the law's passage.

Controlling Costs: The Great Weakness of ObamaCare

The second big goal of ObamaCare — holding down out-of-control medical costs that increase the price of insurance for all Americans — seems much less likely to be achieved in the long term (it obviously has not since the law's passage). As Charles Boorady, a managing director with Credit Suisse, observed at a conference devoted to studying the issue: "Most of us agree [ObamaCare] will probably boost the insured population and you could probably give it an A. But I think it gets an F on bending the cost curve up instead of down."

It's obviously much more difficult to control costs in a free market than it is to simply spend almost a trillion dollars to insure millions of Americans. As the old saying goes, you get what you pay for, and if Americans pay more for healthcare per person than other countries in the developed world, part of the reason is that the quality and quantity of care is higher in this country than in others, at least to those who have full access to the system.

For example, there are more than three times as many Magnetic Resonance Imaging (MRI) devices in the United States per capita as in any other developed nation. The widespread use of advanced medical devices is expensive, but even so few Americans would want to decrease their access to these technologies which help them when their health is at risk and improve the overall quality of their lives.

Critics of the current system nonetheless argue that healthcare in the United States is inferior to that available in many places throughout the world. They typically point out that life expectancy is much shorter here than in Japan, the world leader. In that country people live on average to about 83 years of age while in the United States the average lifespan is about 78 years. About 35 countries fall in between, giving critics of American healthcare ample fodder to make what seems to be a persuasive case that our system lags behind the rest of the world.

Appearances, however, can be deceiving. Yes, compared to Japan's top ranking the U.S. lifespan number looks bad, but this shouldn't obscure another important fact: Americans live much longer than the world average, which is 67 years. In fact, life expectancy in the United States is about at the level of other industrialized nations (the average is 80 years, according to the Organisation for Economic Co-operation and Development).

The five-year gap in lifespan versus the world leader is significant, and we can do better than the current shortfall, but our healthcare system is not the only variable that explains the difference. The Japanese and other people around the world have much healthier lifestyles than Americans do and this fact does much to explain our variance with them.

> **? DID YOU KNOW . . .**
> More than $1 billion in consumer rebates were sent out in 2012 by insurers that failed to meet a new rule, requiring them to spend at least 80-85 cents of every dollar on healthcare – not tied to such expenditures as administrative expenses, overhead or advertising.

It's easy to see this stark difference in lifestyles when we look at the nations that eat the most and exercise the least. According to *Forbes* magazine, the United States is #9 in a ranking of the world's most obese nations (the first eight are mostly Polynesian states like the Cook Islands and Micronesia). Japan, in sharp contrast, ranks #163 out of 194. If the Japanese live five years longer than us it probably has more to do with their healthy diets, higher activity levels and trim physiques than with the quality of their healthcare system, which by all accounts is above average.

This said, there is still much room for improvement in the American healthcare system. The United States currently spends about 17 percent of Gross Domestic Product (GDP) on healthcare — a level that is almost double that of the OECD average and more than twice what it was in 1980, when it stood at 9 percent. The bad news doesn't end there. In 1980, the federal government accounted for about 25 percent of the nation's healthcare spending, while today it has spiked to 45 percent and will continue to grow as the Baby Boomer generation ages over the next 15 years.

It is important to note that many countries with national healthcare like Britain and Canada benefit from the medical innovations and new drugs that emanate from America's profit-driven system. Medical companies and Big Pharma make their money off of American consumers only to sell their products at cheaper prices to state-run systems abroad.

For sure, the healthcare entitlement monster is putting immense pressure on the federal budget, with Medicaid and Medicare today accounting for 21 percent of the government's total outlays. And yet for all the money the United States spends to provide healthcare for its citizens we have an average lifespan that is two years shorter than the OECD. Clearly, the system can be made more cost effective.

There are undoubtedly ways to bend the cost curve down, while still maintaining a system that not only extends life, but improves its quality. The United States performs twice as many knee replacements per capita as the European Union and that costs money, driving up our healthcare expenditures compared to our neighbors across the Atlantic Ocean. But we want to keep this high level because all those extra knee replacements make the lives of our citizens who receive them better.

ObamaCare attempts to deal with the cost issue with our healthcare system, but only in a halfhearted way. The new law's priorities are mostly focused on decreasing the number of the uninsured and increasing consumer benefits — not on holding down costs.

More Benefits Mean Higher Costs

Contrary to the insistence of ObamaCare supporters that the new law bends the cost curve down, it obviously moves it in the opposite direction by imposing an expensive array of new mandates on the insurance industry.

The most important of the new rules prevents insurance companies from rejecting people (or charging them more) because they have a pre-existing health condition, in effect forcing insurers to accept anyone as an enrollee who wants to sign up no matter how much the person is likely to cost in the amount of benefits paid out. In insurance jargon, this is called "guaranteed issue."

Other significant rules prevent insurance companies from capping the amount of benefits they have to pay out over a given year or during a beneficiary's lifetime. Now, when a catastrophic health condition occurs in a policyholder's life an insurance company will be on the hook to cover the beneficiaries' expenses on an unlimited basis. Needless to say, an open-ended stream of benefits in extreme cases could cost a staggering amount of money over the long term.

TAB. 9-1: **IMPACT OF OBAMACARE ON INSURANCE COSTS**	
New ObamaCare Benefit/Regulation	**Pressure On Costs**
No Pre-existing Condition Rejections	
Children Insured On Parents Plans To Age 26	
No Caps on Annual Benefits	↑
No Caps on Lifetime Benefits	
No Rescissions	
"Essential Health Benefits" Must Be Covered	
Tighter "Medical Loss Ratios"	
Restrictions on Premium Discrimination	

Other new rules will also raise costs by preventing insurance companies from canceling insurance policies for frivolous reasons (called "rescissions" in industry jargon) and requiring them to include "essential health benefits" in all their insurance plans.

Under another ObamaCare rule, insurers must maintain tight "medical loss ratios," measuring the share of their revenues that are devoted to medical benefits for policyholders. This rule, which micromanages the budgets of insurers, will restrict their profit margins and encourage them to raise prices to offset lost financial gains. More than $1 billion in consumer rebates were sent out in 2012 by insurers that failed to meet this rule, requiring them to spend at least 80-85 cents of every dollar on healthcare — not tied to such expenditures as administrative expenses, overhead or advertising.

In addition, insurance companies must now cover children up to the age of 26 as dependents (they cannot be charged as adults) on the plans of parents who make this choice. Tighter restrictions are also placed on the amount of premiums that can be charged to different policyholders based on their commitment to prevention and personal wellness.

Why Did the Insurance Industry Support ObamaCare?

ObamaCare imposes new financial burdens on insurance companies, for sure, but we can surmise from the industry's support for the new law that it will — in its totality and over the long term — be good for major insurers. Two big reasons for the insurance industry's backing of ObamaCare:

- First, the new law gives insurers as many as 30 million more customers (this figure assumes all states eventually participate in Medicaid's expansion). This gigantic new market, which is almost as big as the population of Canada, will be compelled by law to buy the industry's products. Many of the newly insured will also be given money by the government to make their purchase, making them ideal customers.

- Secondly, insurance companies remain free to pass along the increased costs that come with the new ObamaCare mandates to their customers in the form of higher premiums, co-pays and deductibles. Insurers could suffer painful consequences if they raise prices too much, such as being prevented from selling insurance through the exchanges, but the new law comes with no explicit price controls.

The addition of as many as 30 million more customers to the health insurance system will probably bring with it economies of scale that eventually lowers costs. But it seems unlikely that this beneficial byproduct of an increased market for insurance will be enough to offset other factors driving up costs.

Are Healthcare Costs Rising Because of ObamaCare?

That, as they say, is the $64,000 question. It's difficult to answer because cause and effect is never simple in a complex marketplace like health insurance, but an increasing preponderance of evidence supports the assertion of ObamaCare critics that costs are indeed rising because of the new law.

In September 2011 the Kaiser Family Foundation reported that health insurance premiums had increased for American families by 9 percent compared to the previous year — the largest spike upward since 2004. This came on top of news that the American Association of Retired Persons (AARP) — the powerful lobby representing the nation's senior citizens — would increase the health insurance premiums of its employees from 8 percent to 13 percent.

The rise in costs could be most clearly seen in the administration's decision to grant non-compliance waivers to many unions and businesses because they threatened to drop their coverage under the additional financial burden generated by new ObamaCare rules.

Unwilling to see the number of uninsured Americans suddenly surge and the new law unravel as a consequence, the White House gladly granted them relief. In doing so, President Obama sidestepped disaster

? DID YOU KNOW . . .

To help adults with pre-existing conditions who are in desperate need of health insurance and can't obtain it before 2014, ObamaCare creates a special pre-existing condition insurance program or temporary "high-risk pool" in each state.

for his healthcare reform package, but he also raised an obvious question in the minds of the many Americans who wondered: "Where's our waiver from ObamaCare?"

We won't be able to fully judge the impact of the new law until its major elements (the expansion of Medicaid and the state-based exchanges) become operational in 2014, but if health insurance costs continue to move upward in coming years, the future of ObamaCare will become increasingly imperiled. The White House can only issue so many non-compliance waivers without undermining the new law. As of the summer of 2012, at least 1,625 waivers had been granted.

A Review of the New ObamaCare Mandates

What exactly are the new ObamaCare mandates that have put so much upward pressure on health insurance costs? Let's go through the most important rules one by one.

NO PRE-EXISTING CONDITION REJECTIONS

It's hard not to sympathize with someone who gets sick and then is denied health insurance because of their condition, but if we look at it from the perspective of the insurance company, we can understand why it happens.

Insurance companies are not charitable organizations. They are in business to make a profit by selling insurance, and insurance — as the word is commonly defined — is financial protection you insulate yourself with before you need it, not something you obtain after the fact.

Buying health insurance for a pre-existing health condition is a little bit like buying fire insurance after your house has already started burning. Any insurance company interested in avoiding bankruptcy would, of course, never sell someone such a policy, but that is exactly what health insurance companies do when they sell policies to Americans with pre-existing conditions.

The ObamaCare ban on denying coverage to children who suffer a pre-existing condition is already operative. It went into effect in September 2010 (plans that have "grandfathered" status, however, are not required to comply with the new rule). The pre-existing condition rule will be expanded to adults in January 2014.

While we wait for that date, the news thus far concerning the new mandate is troubling. Rather than provide this expensive coverage for children who have a pre-existing health condition, many insurers have simply stopped selling child-only insurance plans. The ObamaCare mandate has no power over them if they completely drop out of this market, which it makes no sense for them to compete in if they are guaranteed to lose money in the process.

Although insurers won't be able to do the same when the pre-existing condition mandate is applied to adults in 2014 (they would have to dissolve their businesses to do so), the negative reaction to the mandate as it applies to children suggests significant problems ahead for this new rule. While it undoubtedly will help many needy Americans, it also threatens to undermine the viability of the entire health insurance market.

TEMPORARY "HIGH-RISK POOL" IN EACH STATE

To help adults with pre-existing conditions who are in desperate need of health insurance and can't obtain it before 2014 (when the new rule takes effect for adults), ObamaCare creates a special pre-existing condition insurance program or "temporary high-risk pool" in each state. These government run insurance plans are supported by $5 billion in federal funding in addition to contributions from each state that agrees to participate.

Eligibility to enter the program is limited to American citizens and legal immigrants who have a pre-existing condition and have been uninsured for at least six months. Premium amounts can vary by age, but the amount that older enrollees can be charged is capped at four times the lowest amount paid by anyone else. Deductibles are fixed to the Health Savings Account limits — $5,950 for an individual and $11,900 for a family.

Operative only 90 days after ObamaCare was signed into law, the high-risk pool began enrolling people in August and September 2010. Thus far, it has gotten off to a slow start, which is something of a surprise since critics predicted that the program would be overwhelmed and rapidly run out of money.

Application rates have been extremely low, with only about 8,000 people enrolled nationwide as of November 2010. Seeing that a single state (Pennsylvania) with the lowest premium offered ($283 per month) accounted for the largest number of enrollees (1,650), the program has reduced its prices in every state to help spur enrollment.

Even if more people sign up, low enrollment thus far suggests that the pre-existing condition issue was wildly overblown to help build popular support for ObamaCare as a whole. It obviously is not the dire national crisis it was made out to be.

More than two dozen states now run their own pre-existing condition insurance plans (PCIP) with federal money, while the rest rely on the federal Department of Health and Human Services to administer their plans. To qualify, you must be uninsured for at least six months and be able to provide proof you applied for individual insurance and were denied coverage because of a pre-existing condition. To find a plan, visit the federal government's website at *www.PCIP.gov* or call HHS at 866-717-5826.

CHILDREN CAN BE INSURED ON THEIR PARENTS' PLAN UP TO AGE 26

By allowing children up to the age of 26 who are not married to be covered by their parents' insurance plans, ObamaCare places another significant new cost onto the shoulders of insurance companies as these individuals must be counted as regular dependent children under age 18 and not as adults. This provision of the law took effect in September 2010.

The new rule, however, does not apply in all cases. Retirees under the age of 65 will not be able to use their insurance to cover adult children as dependents. And adult children with a parent already enrolled in Medicare won't be able to stay on their parents' insurance either. Children up to age 26 may also be denied coverage under their parents' plan if they are able to obtain health insurance through their employer.

NO ANNUAL OR LIFETIME CAPS ON BENEFITS

Insurance companies have traditionally held down their costs by capping the amount of money they pay out on claims, limiting the duration of payments to a given year or to some other period of time in a beneficiary's lifetime. ObamaCare eliminates these limits.

The ban on lifetime limits ended in September 2010 for all health insurance plans, even those already in operation (plans with "grandfathered" status are not exempt). As for annual limits, a full ban begins in January 2014. Before that time, the ceiling on annual limits is steadily raised for all employer-based plans and new individual plans as follows:

- September 2010: $750,000

- September 2011: $1,250,000

- September 2012: $2,000,000

- January 2014: No Limit Allowed

> **? DID YOU KNOW . . .**
> Beginning in January 2014 all new insurance plans will be required to include coverage for "essential health benefits."

Although the elimination of time-sensitive caps on insurance benefits is a popular measure, it restricts the choices of American consumers. No longer will they be able to buy bargain-basement insurance plans, which are offered at low prices in part because they include strict limits on the amount of money that can be paid out in benefits.

Although these "Mini-Med" plans are frequently attacked by critics as equivalent to inferior, snake oil insurance, millions of low-income Americans and the businesses they work for have come to rely on the coverage they provide, notwithstanding their deficiencies compared to pricier coverage.

Supporters of ObamaCare generally want to eliminate this market and many, including Senator John D. Rockefeller of West Virginia, were angered when the White House granted non-compliance waivers to companies like McDonald's allowing them to continue "Mini-Med" coverage for their employees. Believing that more than a million Americans are duped by these low-cost plans, Rockefeller asserted that they are "worse than nothing because of the false expectations and the false hope" they set up for consumers, who often find the coverage they need is not actually included in their plan.

NO RESCISSIONS

One of the biggest complaints against insurance companies has been their controversial use of so-called "rescissions" — an unsavory practice used to deny coverage immediately after a person suffers a serious and costly health setback.

Rather than cover legitimate medical costs as promised by contractual agreement, the insurance company cancels the policyholder's entire insurance plan. Often, insurers justify the action by citing a policyholder's misstatements in their insurance contract, even if these are minor, unintentional errors that have nothing to do with the health setback the policyholder needs covered.

As of September 2010 insurers are no longer permitted to cancel the insurance plans of policyholders for these types of frivolous reasons. Although this is obviously the right thing to do (and one of the better parts of ObamaCare), it will no doubt serve to exert upward pressure on the premiums everyone has to pay as insurers are forced to pay out more in benefits than in the past.

Keep in mind that this provision of ObamaCare does not mean that an insurance company can never cancel an individual's policy. If outright fraud has been committed the new rule will not help protect the wrongdoer, who will likely lose his or her coverage as a consequence.

"ESSENTIAL HEALTH BENEFITS" COVERED

Beginning in January 2014 all new insurance plans — whether they are offered through the private, group or exchange markets — will be required to include coverage for "essential health benefits." This rule effectively creates a new national standard for health insurance, raising the quality of coverage for all Americans.

The list of essential health benefits has not yet been decided by the Department of Health and Human Services, but it did release information about the broad areas covered by the list (See Appendix A). We also know that each plan must at the very least cover 60 percent of the medical costs, on average, of its enrollees (i.e., the minimum level of coverage represented by the Bronze plan sold through the exchanges).

While this new rule seems reasonable enough on the surface, it will in conjunction with other ObamaCare rules prevent insurance companies from offering bargain-basement "Mini-Med" plans to consumers, plans that have historically been profitable for them and attractive to many American consumers and businesses.

Mandating "essential health benefits" is a little bit like the government outlawing motorcycles because they offer less protection in an accident than an automobile. Such a requirement would undoubtedly reduce injuries and deaths on the road, but it would also encroach on the choices that Americans have always been free to make for themselves. Many ObamaCare rules make a similar tradeoff in favor of more protection, generating opposition from those who wish to retain the range of choices that have been available to them in the past.

"MEDICAL-LOSS RATIOS" TIGHTENED

In an effort to suppress insurance plans that allocate a large portion of premiums toward non-medical expenses such as administration, marketing, overhead and profits, ObamaCare establishes tighter limits on "medical-loss ratios" or MLR. This metric, expressed as a percentage of an insurance plan's total revenue, is used by the insurance industry to describe how much is paid out directly to policyholders in benefits.

The decision to establish a firm MLR is one of the better aspects of ObamaCare. Back in 1993, a time when many more non-profit insurers existed, the average MLR stood at 95 percent, meaning that the typical insurer paid out 95 cents of every dollar the company took in from premiums for the claims of policy holders. In the 20 years since that time, that level dropped to about 80 percent as non-profit insurers disappeared and Wall Street demanded more and more profit taking.

Not wanting the level to fall even more, ObamaCare creates a new floor. In the large group market where big businesses shop, insurance plans must now spend 85 percent or more of their revenue on the direct medical costs of plan participants, and if they do not, they must reimburse participants with rebates that make up the difference to them.

In the individual and small group markets (where small businesses buy their health insurance), the threshold is set a little lower at 80 percent in deference to the reality that smaller plans have less budget flexibility than bigger plans.

The new ObamaCare MLR thresholds are already in place and many Americans may have noticed unexpectedly receiving rebate checks in the mail from their health insurance provider. In total, almost 13 million people have received about $1.1 billion from insurers who generated MLRs that fell below the new thresholds.

Failure to comply with the new rule could trigger even more painful consequences for insurers than merely having to send out rebate checks to their policyholders. If an insurance plan does not meet the ObamaCare threshold for three straight years, it could be prevented from selling policies to new customers. If it fails to meet it for five straight years the Department of Health and Human Services could terminate the insurance plan's contract with all of its existing policyholders.

Needless to say, the new rule governing medical loss ratios is one of the most unpleasant parts of ObamaCare for the insurance industry to swallow. It is a new rule that has not received the attention it deserves.

What exactly constitutes a "direct medical expense"? That is still something of an open question. Insurers, of course, want the broadest interpretation possible to give them more flexibility to manage their balance sheets. Consumer groups, in contrast, want a narrow interpretation so that more money is paid out in insurance benefits to policyholders.

To balance these competing interests, the new law directed the National Association of Insurance Commissioners (NAIC) to establish the criteria that would be used to determine what was and what was not a "direct medical expense." The Commission issued its report in October 2010, which the Department of Health and Human Services is expected to certify and eventually make operative. Here are a few of the NAIC's more important rulings:

- **Aggregating Costs Across State Lines** — Insurers wanted to be able to calculate their medical-loss ratios using regions of the country as large as possible so that they could even out their expenses as needed. The NAIC recommended that they could not do this, requiring them to calculate their ratios only within a given state.

> ❓ **DID YOU KNOW . . .**
>
> **Under ObamaCare, insurers will no longer be able to reject people because of a pre-existing health condition, nor will they be able to charge people higher premiums if they have one.**

- **Federal Taxes Excluded** — Although the new law directly states that "federal and state taxes and licensing or regulatory fees" should be excluded when medical loss ratios are calculated, Congressional Democrats insisted that this referred only to taxes imposed specifically by ObamaCare. In a victory for the insurance industry, the NAIC ruled that the language of the law should be interpreted to mean all federal taxes, including income taxes, but not taxes on investment gains. If this

NAIC ruling remains in force insurers will have an easier time reaching the medical loss ratios required by law. As such, it's a victory for them.

- **Year-to-Year Fluctuations** — Small insurance companies, in particular, were worried that they would have difficulty reaching a consistent 80 percent medical-loss ratio every year because of natural fluctuations in their business over extended periods of time. Some years they might pay out a large amount in benefits and in others the amount could be relatively small as revenues grow to be used against future outlays. Receptive to this argument, the NAIC recommended that credits called "credibility adjustments" be given to small insurers to help them even out temporary imbalances.

- **Fraud Control and Utilization Review** — Insurers wanted their attempts to limit fraud and their internal reviews, in which they decided whether or not to cover specific medical treatments, to be excluded from their medical loss ratio calculation. The NAIC ruled against them.

When issuing these rulings the NAIC stated that the formula for calculating medical loss ratios was not something that should be considered set in stone. It said that the formula should evolve over time to reflect the realities of the marketplace. If, for instance, the formula proved an unreasonable hardship for insurance companies, it might have to be loosened.

Critics of ObamaCare argue that the medical loss ratios established by the new law will effectively push small insurance companies (which typically have low medical loss ratios because they must pay more for administrative costs and the like than large insurance companies) out of the market. If that happened it would decrease the level of overall competition and put upward pressure on insurance prices. But it's more likely that the ratio would be adjusted down for small insurers if such an action were needed to protect their position in the market.

RESTRICTIONS ON PREMIUM DISCRIMINATION

Under ObamaCare, insurers will no longer be able to reject people because of a pre-existing health condition, nor will they be able to charge people higher premiums if they have one. The new law prevents most other types of price discrimination by stipulating that premiums within a health insurance plan can only be different person-to-person based on an individual's:

- **Age** (premiums for older people cannot be more than three times as much than for younger people)

- **Tobacco usage** (smokers can be charged higher premiums)

- **Geographic location** (policyholders that live in a part of the state or region with a high cost of living can be charged more)

While the effect of these non-discrimination rules will protect some policyholders from higher prices, it is likely to shift insurance costs to the entire pool of plan participants and increase premiums for everyone enrolled. In effect, it forces low-risk individuals to subsidize the health insurance of high-risk individuals. An obese, couch potato, for example, will pay no more than one who is svelte and exercises regularly, everything else being equal between them.

RIGHT TO APPEAL

Although its impact on insurance costs will likely be negligible, one other ObamaCare rule is worth mentioning. If you get into a dispute with your insurance company, you'll be able to seek an outside review by a government agency. Some states already allow such reviews, but now you'll be able to do this throughout the entire country.

The infrastructure is not yet in place to deal with appeals everywhere, but by 2014 it should be. Anyone still may choose to challenge his or her insurance company's decisions through the legal system.

WILL OBAMACARE RULES APPLY TO MY CURRENT HEALTH INSURANCE PLAN?

President Obama repeatedly promised both during his campaign for office and once he entered the White House that Americans would be able to keep their health insurance. To help follow through on that promise the new law stipulates that plans that were in operation prior to March 23, 2010, (the day ObamaCare became law) could be "grandfathered," that is to say exempted from most of the new rules and regulations.

While this sounds great, the finer points in the provision drain it of real power. If you're enrolled in your employer's insurance plan, for instance, it's up to the company to determine whether or not it wants grandfathered status. According to the Robert Wood Johnson Foundation only 35 percent of employers are expected to make this choice.

That's because under the new law employers can only keep their grandfathered status if they agree not to change their plans in other ways. For example, if a plan raises its premiums, drops some benefit or changes its insurance carrier, it will immediately lose its grandfathered status.

Whatever employers choose, they must notify their employees whether or not their insurance plan will be grandfathered or not. Intent on maintaining the flexibility to manage their plans, most employers will probably choose to comply with the new ObamaCare rules. Because of this likelihood it's fair to say that President Obama's promise that you can keep your current insurance will prove hollow in the end, an unintended consequence of the new law.

TURNING THE SCREWS ON MEDICARE

10

MEDICARE IS ONE OF THE MOST IMPORTANT components of the nation's healthcare system, providing coverage for the oldest Americans (all citizens age 65 and over can join the program), who also happen to be the group that needs the most care. Toward that end the federal government spent $528 billion to support the program in 2010 — a level expected to rise above $1 trillion by 2020.

Given the ocean of money funding Medicare it was inevitable that the authors of ObamaCare would tap into it to pay for the new healthcare system. As a consequence, senior citizens suffer the biggest financial blow from the new law. That's because Medicare's budget is cut by about $45 billion per year on average over the next decade.

In an effort to mask the bad taste of this medicine ObamaCare throws Medicare recipients a bone by improving their prescription drug coverage, but this gesture does not begin to make up for hundreds of billions in lost revenue. Still, it's something positive that seniors can welcome. Let's take a closer look at this sliver of good news before we move on to the budget cuts that cloud Medicare's future.

Closing the "Donut Hole"

Very few younger Americans have probably ever heard of the "donut hole" in Medicare's prescription drug program, but if you're on Medicare and need expensive drugs it's likely you have. Medicare recipients typically pay a deductible of a few hundred dollars and then 25 percent of the cost of the drugs they need up to a certain point (typically around $2,800 in a person's drug spending). That's when the infamous "donut hole" opens up and recipients have to pay 100 percent of the cost of their drugs up until they reach $6,400 in drug spending. Beyond that amount, insurance coverage kicks in again to close the hole with the recipient paying only 5 percent of drug costs above $6,400.

TAB. 10-1: MEDICARE'S DRUG COVERAGE GAP BEFORE OBAMACARE			
Drug Spending	**Coverage Gap**	**You Pay**	**Medicare Pays**
$0 to $2,800		25%	75%
$2,800 to $6,400	"Donut Hole"	100%	0%
Above $6,400		5%	95%

? DID YOU KNOW . . .

Means testing will expand under Medicare, so that individuals with an income of $85,000 or higher and couples with an income of $170,000 or higher will receive a reduced subsidy that will increase the price they pay for their prescriptions.

Why does this coverage gap exist? As you might expect, the answer has to do with politics. When the legislation creating the Medicare prescription drug program was passed in 2003, limiting coverage in this way was part of a cost-saving compromise that became necessary for the law to gain congressional approval.

Although most people on Medicare never fall into the "donut hole" because their drug expenses don't rise high enough, ObamaCare includes a plan to close it gradually over the next decade and help those who do. To accomplish that goal President Obama and Democratic leaders in Congress made a deal with the pharmaceutical industry, which agreed to subsidize part of the cost of the expanded drug coverage.

Here's how it works. In 2010 Medicare recipients who reached the "donut hole" received a $250 rebate to help reduce their costs. Starting in 2011 help from Big Pharma arrives, with the industry paying 50 percent of the cost of all brand-name drugs (recipients pay the remaining 50 percent). By 2013 the federal government will step in and provide an additional subsidy. This will be phased in over time and by 2020 will cover 25 percent of the cost of brand-name drugs, with Medicare recipients on the hook by that time for only 25 percent when the Big Pharma discount of 50 percent is factored in.

TAB. 10-2: CLOSING THE "DONUT HOLE": NEW REBATES TO HELP PAY THE COST OF BRAND-NAME DRUGS			
Year	You Pay	Drug Company Discount	Government Subsidy
2010	100% but you get a $250 Rebate		
2011	50%	50%	0%
2013	50%	50%	Phase-In Begins
2020	25%	50%	25%

The story is similar for generic drugs except that there is no Big Pharma discount (generic drugs by definition are not owned or manufactured by a single company). Because of this the federal government will do more of the heavy lifting than it does for brand-name drugs, but the result will be the same for Medicare recipients. By 2020 they will only have to pay 25 percent of the cost of generic drugs they buy in the "donut hole" range, the same they will pay for brand-name drugs.

TAB. 10-3: CLOSING THE "DONUT HOLE": NEW REBATES TO HELP PAY THE COST OF BRAND-NAME DRUGS			
Year	You Pay	Drug Company Discount	Government Subsidy
2010	100% but you get a $250 Rebate		
2011	< 100%	0%	Phase-In Begins
2013	< 100%	0%	↓
2020	25%	0%	75%

More Retirees May Need to Use Medicare's Prescription Drugs

One unforeseen consequence of ObamaCare emerged soon after the passage of the law when a group of companies began to drop prescription drug coverage for their retirees. They took this action because the new law, in a misguided effort to raise revenue to fund ObamaCare, eliminated a key tax break that incentivized companies to give their retirees this benefit. Rather than pay more to the federal government the affected companies simply decided to drop their drug coverage for retirees, forcing them onto Medicare's prescription drug plan. If this trend continues, a few million retirees across the country could wind up in the same position.

Means Testing: Lower Subsidies for High-Income Recipients

The other news in Medicare's prescription drug plan involves the expansion of means testing. Such testing already exists for high-income recipients as part of other parts of Medicare and now it will function in a similar way with the prescription drug plan. Specifically, individuals with an income of $85,000 or higher and couples with an income of

$170,000 or higher will receive a reduced subsidy that will increase the price they pay for their prescriptions.

Medicare Spending Cuts

The closure of the "donut hole" is a nice benefit for Medicare recipients, but it shouldn't obscure the more important fact that a huge amount of the revenue needed to fund ObamaCare will come directly out of Medicare's budget. According to the Congressional Budget Office — the non-partisan government agency that makes budgetary forecasts — roughly 42 percent of the total $1 trillion dollar cost of ObamaCare will come from cuts in Medicare spending over the next decade.

TAB. 10-4: HOW MEDICARE SPENDING CUTS FUND OBAMACARE (2010-2019)		
Total Cost Of ObamaCare And How It's Paid For...	Billions $	Share of Cost
Medicare Spending Cuts	$455	42.3%
Medicare Payment Rate Cuts	$196	18.2%
Medicare Advantage Cuts	$136	12.7%
Other Medicare/Medicaid Cuts	$123	11.4%
Other Revenue Sources	$620	57.7%

Source: Congressional Budget Office

Although President Obama and Congressional Democrats have downplayed the impact of these cuts, stating that they will not affect the quality of care Medicare provides, no one really knows for sure what will happen once spending decreases. One thing seems likely: With the federal government cutting almost a half-trillion dollars from a program that millions of senior citizens rely on, at least some recipients are going to feel it.

The biggest cuts in Medicare will come in two main areas: a reduction in payment rates to providers and a reduction in payment rates to Medicare Advantage plans. Let's look at each in turn.

Medicare Payment Rate Cuts

About one-fifth of the funding for ObamaCare (or $196 billion) will come from cuts to Medicare's payment rates to providers other than physicians over the next 10 years. Money generated by this payment reduction will be redirected toward new healthcare priorities such as the expansion of Medicaid and subsidies for the health insurance exchanges. The people who will feel the pinch the most will be those who currently receive this money, namely providers such as hospitals, skilled nursing facilities, and home health agencies who provide the care that Medicare recipients have come to expect.

Critics of ObamaCare have pointed out that providers could revolt against cuts in their pay and choose not to accept Medicare patients. If that happens, Medicare could become weakened by a phenomenon that has plagued the Medicaid program for years: the refusal of doctors and facilities to participate. As it stands today, private insurance already pays more than Medicare on a per-patient basis and more doctors and providers may be pushed by the reductions to turn to that higher paying source.

What does this mean for you? If you're on Medicare you may have to find a new doctor or wait longer for appointments with your current doctor because he or she has more Medicare patients to care for. It also could mean that the quality of doctors who serve Medicare patients decreases on average, lowering the quality of care you are accustomed to receiving. Certain facilities may also be less receptive to caring for Medicare beneficiaries.

Medicare Advantage Cuts

All Medicare recipients are likely to feel the effects of a reduction in payment rates to providers, but those who are enrolled in the Medicare Advantage program (about one in four) will feel additional pain. According to the Congressional Budget Office these senior citizens will get about $68 less a month in Medicare Advantage benefits because of ObamaCare.

The Medicare Advantage program was designed to open up Medicare to private insurers like Cigna Health Insurance, Aetna Inc. and UnitedHealthcare with the goal of controlling costs as managed care plans had for many U.S. employers. It was thought that outside insurers would make better use of tax dollars than government bureaucrats while simultaneously providing senior citizens with additional benefits beyond their standard Medicare coverage.

Senior citizens usually need more than basic Medicare, which only covers about 60 percent of their medical expenses on average. Those with the financial means buy so-called "Medigap" coverage as a supplement, but those with lower incomes do not have this option. That's where Medicare Advantage comes in, giving government financial assistance to help lower-income senior citizens secure additional coverage. This additional coverage can include beneficiaries enjoying reduced co-payments or coinsurance for services that the traditional Medicare program covers, but it can also include coverage for services such as hearing aids or gym memberships that Medicare does not normally cover.

> **"We know that cuts in Medicare are being used to fund national healthcare reform. And we also had concerns about our ability to build a network of healthcare providers that would meet the needs of our seniors."**
> — Lynn Bowman, a vice president of Harvard Pilgrim

In cutting Medicare Advantage's spending, ObamaCare ironically enough turns its guns on millions of low-income Americans — the people it's supposedly committed to helping. How did that happen? Congressional Democrats, seizing on a report that found that private insurance companies were not spending enough of their government-provided Medicare Advantage money on "direct medical expenses," singled it out as a target for cuts. The program, in short, had an unacceptably low "medical loss ratio" which suggested that private insurers were making excessive profits at the expense of taxpayers.

To eliminate this inefficient use of taxpayer money, ObamaCare cuts $136 billion dollars out of the Medicare Advantage budget over the next 10 years. Some insurers in the program will be hurt more than others, depending on how well they use taxpayer dollars (i.e., those with strong medical loss ratios will be protected from penalties and in some cases even rewarded). The impact on insurers will also vary by geographic location, depending on different performance standards established by counties within each state.

How does this affect participants in the program? The private insurance companies that are part of Medicare Advantage will likely cut benefits and/or raise premiums. The insurers could also find the changes too much to bear and leave Medicare Advantage altogether. Something that had been observed previously when payment rates to Medicare managed care plans were reduced.

That has already begun to happen. In late 2010 Harvard Pilgrim Health Care dropped Medicare Advantage, forcing 22,000 senior citizens in New England to look elsewhere to supplement their basic Medicare benefits. It did so because of reduced reimbursements and new rules that required it to create a network of doctors who would, on the whole, charge lower fees.

As Lynn Bowman, a vice president of Harvard Pilgrim, said when explaining the company's decision: "We became concerned by the long-term viability of Medicare Advantage programs in general. We know that cuts in Medicare are being used to fund national healthcare reform. And we also had concerns about our ability to build a network of healthcare providers that would meet the needs of our seniors."

If other insurers take similar action, the Medicare Advantage program could be seriously undermined and its seven million enrollees could be forced out of the program. Those who remain will have to live with fewer benefits.

Independent Payment Advisory Board (IPAB)

One of the biggest obstacles to reform under our system of government is the lack of political will needed to pass unpopular laws. Afraid to cast controversial votes that could cost them election victories, political leaders often push difficult public policy problems down the road to the next generation of Americans. Healthcare, of course, is a prominent example of buck-passing as Medicare and Medicaid have proven largely impervious to needed budgetary reform since they were created in the 1960s.

In order to break through this political logjam, ObamaCare will establish a new Independent Payment Advisory Board (IPAB) as a means to reduce healthcare costs in Medicare, a budgetary black hole that sucks in an increasing stream of taxpayer dollars as the American population ages. Although little attention has been paid to the IPAB, it's potentially a powerful cost-cutting mechanism within the new law. Pete Orszag, the former White House budget director, observed that it could be the most important part of ObamaCare in bending the cost curve down.

The new board won't be a rubber stamp on the wishes of the White House and Congress as it will operate independent of their control. Former Senator Tom Daschle, one of ObamaCare's most important architects, tellingly declared in his 2008 book Critical: "The Federal Health Board I envision for our country would be modeled on the U.S. Federal Reserve System." Daschle spent 50 pages explaining why he thought an entity like the IPAB was a good idea.

Daschle got what he wanted. Unlike typical presidential commissions, which usually have no real power, the IPAB will be able to make recommendations that actually mean something. That's because the board's decisions are automatically binding unless Congress blocks them. And that will be difficult to do since the new law stipulates that it will require a three-fifths "super majority" to overturn IPAB decisions (i.e., a filibuster, which requires 60 votes in the Senate, cannot be used). Given this significant hurdle, it seems likely that many of the board's decisions will become the law of the land.

While an empowered, energetic IPAB will create needed budgetary reforms outside the normal legislative process (depending on the reform that could be a good thing), critics see it as another heavy-handed power grab used by ObamaCare to increase government control over of the nation's healthcare system. They argue that the people's elected representatives will be bypassed and spending cuts in Medicare's budget will be handed down as autocratic decrees from appointed healthcare commissars. Those who support the IPAB point out that its undemocratic traits are hardly unprecedented since the Federal Reserve has operated since 1913 without direct political control over its decisions.

However the IPAB is characterized, no one will be able to say that its decisions lack substance. It will consist of a heavyweight panel of 15 experts chosen from academia, think tanks and the healthcare industry. Appointees will be handpicked by the president and must be approved by the Senate before they can take their seat. They'll be asked to make cost-cutting recommendations for Medicare whenever spending per person in the program rises faster than the Consumer Price Index, something which seems likely to occur more often than not.

The Republican Party has expressed a desire to eliminate the board before it gets started. Even if the IPAB convenes, Congress could neutralize its power by stripping away its funding.

If the Republicans attempt to eliminate the IPAB, they will have powerful allies as Big Pharma (the Pharmaceutical Research and Manufacturing Association), hospitals (the American Hospital Association), and doctors (the American Medical Association) have all declared their opposition to it. The American people are also likely to take a dim view of the IPAB once they learn more about it because an influential government body unaccountable to their wishes is contrary to our constitutional guarantee of self-government, the example of the Federal Reserve notwithstanding.

Assuming the board actually begins to operate, it will be able to make binding recommendations starting in 2015 with none implemented until 2018.

COST-CONTROL EXPERIMENTS 11

I N DECREASING THE UNINSURED POPULATION and in guaranteeing a raft of new consumer benefits, ObamaCare is far from restrained. But when it comes to bending the cost curve down, it is hesitant and halting, preferring to push politically charged actions into the future by using a commission such as the Independent Payment Advisory Board.

This kick-the-can-down-the-road approach is evident in an array of pilot programs that are included in the new law. These programs are, in effect, a series of non-binding experiments to test new ways to deliver, manage and pay for healthcare in the United States. That is all well and good, but it doesn't do anything meaningful to deal with the pressing problem of rising costs, which has been exacerbated by new ObamaCare rules.

The pilot programs contain ObamaCare's biggest ideas for the future of healthcare in the United States. The thinking is that if one of these approaches works on a small scale it can be expanded to the entire country. In other words, the new law throws a bunch of ideas up against a wall to see if any stick. In this sense,

? DID YOU KNOW . . .
ObamaCare tests a new demonstration project in Medicare wherein a team of health professionals delivers care to needy Medicare recipients in their own homes.

it's reminiscent of Franklin Roosevelt's "New Deal," which also included many experiments in search of a solution to a pressing national problem.

"Bundled Payments" in Medicare

In light of the huge amount of money that Medicare spends on hospital and post-hospital treatment (more than $200 billion a year), ObamaCare explores new ways to get more value out of taxpayer dollars that are directed at this important area of the healthcare system. It does so by creating a pilot program within Medicare that moves away from the traditional fee-for-service payment model in widespread use today and tests a bundled-payment system for inpatient hospital services and post-discharge treatment.

Under the new scheme a single lump-sum payment will be delivered to an organization such as a hospital, which will then hire a team of healthcare professionals to provide care to an individual patient for a specific health-related "episode" over a set period of time. An episode timeline could, for example, begin three days before hospitalization and end 30 days after discharge. The team might include professionals from the hospital, doctors in a physician group, members of a skilled nursing facility and caregivers in a home healthcare agency.

Bundled payments are one way in which ObamaCare tries to reduce the number of hospital stays by Medicare recipients — a significant factor of driving up costs. As it now stands, a hospital will usually wash its hands of a patient after discharge. The goal of the new pilot program is to prevent such costly breaks in what should ideally be a continuous chain of care. It tries to keep all stakeholders connected to one another throughout the patient's health-related episode regardless of its duration. It also aims to reduce the number of costly hospital readmissions.

The pilot program is scheduled to begin in January 2013 and run for approximately three years. If it proves successful in reducing hospitalizations, as well as the cost of overall care without sacrificing quality, Congress will consider expanding the program. Its performance will be assessed by the Agency for Healthcare Research and Quality (AHRQ), which will use measures such as hospital readmission rates and feedback from patients to make a recommendation to Congress about the program's future viability.

Time will tell whether the pilot test of bundled payments for continuous treatment works, but the new approach would seem on its face to create an incentive for the members of the treatment team to cut corners and skimp on care. After all, the more treatment they provide, the more their profit margins shrink since the amount they are paid is fixed at a specific amount. To help reduce this possibility, members of a treatment team will receive increased financial rewards if they can help patients recover quickly.

> **"The most important contributor to the high cost of U.S. healthcare is over-utilization."**
> — Dr. Ezekiel Emanuel

A bundled-payments system would probably work best when there are no surprises in treatment along the way as with standard, easily defined and managed procedures such as joint replacements. If the system is eventually rolled out across the United States its use might be restricted to medical conditions such as these and avoided for less predictable health conditions.

"Independence At Home" Demonstration

With similar goals in mind, ObamaCare tests a new demonstration project in Medicare wherein a team of health professionals delivers care to needy Medicare recipients in their own homes. If the members of the treatment team are able to prevent hospital readmissions, reduce costs and improve outcomes, all while simultaneously achieving patient satisfaction, they will be given financial rewards.

The program is directed primarily at Medicare recipients who suffer from more than one chronic condition, who have the worst medical outcomes and who cost the most money. It's modeled on similar programs that have proved successful throughout the country.

It's also worth mentioning that the "Independence at Home" demonstration will evaluate "e-care" technology (including remote monitoring of health conditions such as blood pressure by computers and other electronic devices) to see if it helps reduce cost and improve efficiency of care. The program began in January 2012.

"THE PERFECT STORM OF OVERUTILIZATION"

If we want to understand the overarching theme of ObamaCare's experiments in healthcare cost control, it's spelled out in an essay written by President Obama's healthcare adviser, Dr. Ezekiel Emanuel, in the June 2008 issue of the *Journal of the American Medical Association*.

In his essay titled "The Perfect Storm of Overutilization," Dr. Emanuel asserts that "the most important contributor to the high cost of U.S. healthcare is over-utilization." Too much money he says is spent per person because Americans overuse the healthcare system, visiting doctors and hospitals more than they need to, seeking out expensive specialists in lieu of primary care physicians, and demanding tests and procedures that they don't really need. Higher costs also come because Americans demand amenities such as expensive hospital rooms they could do without. According to Dr. Emanuel the way to control healthcare costs is to wring fluffy, self-indulgent excess out of the system.

Part of this excess he says comes from the current fee-for-service payment system, which "creates a big incentive for overutilization." Knowing that they will be paid more if they do more, doctors inevitably order more tests and schedule more patient visits than are needed. Fear of malpractice suits may also motivate doctors to prescribe additional and unnecessary tests and procedures. Dr. Emanuel concludes by saying that "costs cannot be controlled unless over-utilization is substantially reduced" by giving better financial incentives to doctors to deliver less care to their patients.

While reducing "overutilization" may seem like a sensible solution, the economist Thomas Sowell has pointed out that spending less on something isn't the same thing as lowering its cost. If, for example, Americans are compelled by ObamaCare to make less use of expensive medical technologies, they will merely do without those technologies and the quality of their care will decrease. The price to use the technologies will remain unchanged.

The debate over "overutilization" ultimately boils down to who decides what constitutes excess and what is truly essential to treat a patient. While sensible rules can be put in place to govern these care decisions in a general sense, doctors are obviously better equipped than government bureaucrats to make treatment decisions for individual patients.

Hospital Readmission Reduction

In another pilot program, again aimed at keeping patients out of hospitals where costs typically rocket upward, ObamaCare tests a pay-for-performance Medicare payment system for hospitals based on readmission levels. It is estimated that about 20 percent of all Medicare patients discharged from hospitals must be readmitted within 30 days, in many cases because they were discharged prematurely because their care was mishandled. The pilot program addresses this problem, which costs Medicare billions of dollars in wasted spending each year, by penalizing hospitals that are the worst offenders.

The Department of Health and Human Services will identify hospitals that have shown weakness in this area and single them out for lower Medicare payments. The goal will be to see if increased accountability for readmissions improves the performance of hospitals in this aspect of care. Isolated hospitals in rural communities or in other areas like inner cities where they are the sole providers of medical services will be excluded from penalties.

Accountable Care Organizations

In another pilot program, ObamaCare encourages the use of so-called Accountable Care Organizations (ACOs), which are groups of healthcare professionals that deliver team-based care to patients similar to that provided in the bundled-payments pilot and the "Independence At Home" demonstration initiatives. ACOs with at least 5,000 Medicare recipients will be able to participate in a demonstration program created by the new law. Each ACO that signs up must accept all patients, even those in the worst health.

The program will work this way: Hospitals, physicians and home-care providers will work together to deliver comprehensive and continuous care to each patient that agrees to participate. Each member of the treatment team will be paid by the government on a fee-for-service basis, with bonuses paid out for quality care that is delivered below a given dollar threshold (these have yet to be determined by the Department of Health and Human Services). The idea is to provide an incentive to each member of the treatment team to cooperate and drive down costs. The program began in January 2012 and lasts three years.

The authors of ObamaCare believe that Accountable Care Organizations are the future of healthcare delivery in the United States. If they're right, the cost of care will decrease with the expansion of ACOs throughout the country. Although the ACO pilot program is only a small part of ObamaCare, it is central to the new law's underlying, long-term objective: abolish the fragmented healthcare system currently in use today and replace it with networks of doctors, specialists and hospitals working together in efficient, coordinated harmony.

Accountable Care Organizations are in a general sense analogous to the health insurance exchanges that will be set up in each state in 2014. The exchanges are designed to be great magnets pulling different types of health insurance under their umbrellas. They will start out as marketplaces for insurance sold to individuals and small businesses, but eventually they could absorb the entire employer-based insurance system that is used today by half of the American population.

ACOs are in a much earlier stage of development than the exchanges, but they are also meant to function as great magnets, pulling in healthcare professionals the same way the exchanges pull in individuals and businesses. Both ACOs and the exchanges promise, in short, to centralize healthcare in the United States in order to make it cheaper and better. This isn't quite socialized medicine, but it is a step in that direction.

ObamaCare's requirement that the nation's Medicare program create an ACO program is well under way. As of mid-2012, 154 individual ACOs had been approved by the White House and are in operation serving about 2.4 million Medicare patients. They are expected to save as much as $5 billion over the next eight years. ACOs are also sprouting up in the private sector with doctor groups, hospitals and private insurers leading the way instead of the federal government. Blue Shield of California, for instance, has six ACOs currently operating in the state.

> **? DID YOU KNOW . . .**
> One of the biggest reasons for rising medical costs in the United States is the high prices doctors must pay for medical malpractice insurance. According to an analysis by the journal *Health Affairs*, $56 billion (2.4% of all healthcare spending) is spent on medical malpractice insurance each year.

Comparative Effectiveness Research

ObamaCare promises to eventually bring down healthcare costs in the United States by leveraging best practices as seen in pilot programs funded by the new law. To achieve the same end it also promises to make heavy use of so-called "comparative effectiveness research," which is a fancy way of saying that the government will study the hard data associated with healthcare delivery to determine where the greatest savings can be made and where the system can be improved most.

In this effort ObamaCare will certainly not lack information as study after study produced by academia, think tanks, foundations and the like have shown that the current healthcare system generates massive waste and overspending.

To supervise its comparative effectiveness research, ObamaCare will create a non-profit Patient Centered Outcomes Research Institute. The institute will be managed by a board of governors and its findings will be used as non-binding recommendations. A more powerful agency like the Independent Payment Advisory Board, however, will be free to act on its findings.

WHAT ABOUT TORT REFORM?

One of the biggest reasons for rising medical costs in the United States is the high prices doctors must pay for medical malpractice insurance. According to an analysis by the journal *Health Affairs*, a massive amount of money ($56 billion or 2.4 percent of all healthcare spending) is spent on medical malpractice insurance each year.

No doctor wants to be on the hook for millions of dollars if he or she makes a mistake, causes a patient harm and loses a lawsuit. As a result, many doctors practice "defensive medicine," ordering more tests than they need to and undertaking procedures that are not necessary to reduce their legal jeopardy.

The impact of defensive medicine can be clearly seen, for example, in the high number of babies born by Caesarean section, many of which result not from medical need but rather from doctors wanting to protect themselves from a potential lawsuit.

Although ObamaCare is rooted in the idea that overutilization drives up medical costs (and defensive medicine practices indisputably add fuel to this fire), the new law does almost nothing in the area of tort reform. It does award grants to the states over a five-year period to study alternatives to medical litigations, but this is lip service given to the issue, not real action. According to President Obama's first budget director, Pete Orzag, the new law "missed an important opportunity to shield from malpractice liability any doctors who followed evidence-based guidelines in treating their patients."

In supporting tort reform, Orzag went off the reservation and joined many critics of ObamaCare, but his argument was different from theirs. The critics usually support capping the amount of damages that can be awarded in medical malpractice lawsuits. Orzag, in contrast, supports the idea of creating safe harbors for doctors who follow approved practices and standards based on hard evidence.

Whatever the best approach to tort reform is, ObamaCare opens itself up for just criticism by harping on "overutilization" as a central problem of the current healthcare system and then turning around and doing nothing to discourage defensive medicine — one of its most significant drivers. The charge of conservatives that President Obama and his party were more concerned with placating their supporters — the trial lawyers, who get rich on fat legal settlements and jury awards — than in sincerely seeking to fix the healthcare system is strengthened by the glaring inconsistency within ObamaCare between loud over-utilization complaints and complete tort reform silence.

PART IV

OBAMACARE: THE FINE PRINT

"Beyond federal oversight, ObamaCare includes specific provisions to move us closer to the end goal of being healthier as a nation."

MAKING AMERICANS HEALTHIER 12

I F YOU PAID ATTENTION during the national debate over ObamaCare before it became law, you might think that President Obama's healthcare reform agenda was concerned only with government takeover of the nation's healthcare system and "death panels" deciding end-of-life questions for individuals. These were and are important issues, for sure, but the finished law is about more than its most controversial components.

While few have noticed, ObamaCare includes a new initiative designed to help Americans live healthier lives. It creates a "National Prevention, Health Promotion and Public Health Council" to help manage the government's efforts to promote personal wellness. The council will spend a year or more reviewing the subject and issue a report with recommendations on how to improve the overall health of the American people in order to help them avoid serious health conditions.

Beyond federal oversight, ObamaCare includes specific provisions to move us closer to the end goal of being healthier as a nation. These include:

- No co-pays for approved preventive tests (these are now guaranteed as "essential health benefits" and include things like mammograms and colonoscopies)

- Approval of and support for employer-based programs that reward employees for personal wellness

- Nutritional labeling for food served in restaurants

- Increased spending in Medicaid for preventive services

- Prevention counseling in Medicare

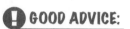 **GOOD ADVICE:**

The Department of Health and Human Services will determine "essential health benefits" that must be covered by insurance plans. To check which tests currently receive the highest federal ratings, visit *http://epss.ahrq.gov.* See Appendix A for more information about the essential health benefits list.

No Co-Pays for Approved Preventive Services

Signaling its intention to take prevention seriously, ObamaCare requires insurance plans — both those on the private market and those sold through the exchanges — to cover the cost of government-approved preventive services such as breast cancer screenings and cholesterol tests. This means that plan participants can no longer be charged co-pays when they want to have one of these tests conducted.

Plans with "grandfathered" status, however, will be exempted from the new requirement, which apply to all insurance plans from January 1, 2011, onward regardless of when a participant enrolled.

ObamaCare's controversial mandate requiring all insurers to make contraception available to women has been made under the law's provision that preventive services be made available without co-pays. The Catholic Church has challenged this rule, arguing that pregnancy is not a disease that needs to be prevented, but rather a normal and necessary condition that women experience at times to perpetuate the existence of humanity.

Prevention as a Guaranteed "Essential Health Benefit"

The Department of Health and Human Services has yet to determine the specific preventive tests that must be covered by insurance plans going forward, but eventually it will publish a list of procedures that are part of a package of "essential health benefits" (see Appendix A for the November 2012 announcement by HHS).

In creating the list of approved preventive procedures, the Health and Human Services Secretary will be aided by the U.S. Preventive Services Task Force (USPSTF) — a governmental body that evaluates and rates the effectiveness of different preventive tests.

Tests that receive a grade of "A" or "B" are deemed to be particularly effective and therefore recommended to all Americans or to those belonging to appropriate demographic groups. Under the new law, all preventive procedures receiving these "A" or "B" stamps of approval must be covered by insurance plans without co-pays.

TAB. 12-1: U.S. PREVENTIVE SERVICES TASK FORCE RATINGS		
Grade	Provide This Service?	Its Benefit Is...
A	Always	Substantial
B	Always	Moderate to Substantial
C	Not Routinely	Helpful for some
D	Never	None & could be harmful
I	Open Question	Insuffient evidence to judge

The power of the USPSTF comes not only through the preventive tests it recommends, but also through those it does not. This negative power — the ability to steer Americans away from specific tests — generated controversy during the national debate over ObamaCare when the task force ruled that women under the age of 50 no longer needed to get mammograms to screen for breast cancer.

This declaration, stoking fears among many who were already concerned that ObamaCare would ultimately end in the rationing of medical services, unleashed a wave of angry criticism that fell on President Obama and Democrats with a loud thud.

Although the controversy was quickly defused when a special provision was inserted into the final law that said younger women would still be able to get mammograms included with their coverage, it highlighted the potential for similar flareups in the future. Whenever government limits or restricts the access of Americans to specific healthcare procedures it is bound to upset people who value those procedures, even if they only represent the viewpoint of a small minority.

To give a flavor of the tests which will eventually be covered, here is a list of prominent tests that currently receive the USPSTF's highest ratings. For those interested in learning more about whether a specific procedure is covered, the full list can be found on the task force's website at ***http://epss.ahrq.gov*** (the Agency for Healthcare Research and Quality).

TAB. 12-2: **PREVENTION PROCEDURES RECEIVING "A" OR "B" RATING BY USPSTF**	
Procedure	**Group Recommended For**
Aspirin to Prevent Heart Disease	**Men 45-99, Women 55-79**
Cervical Cancer Screening	**Sexually active women**
Colorectal Cancer Screening	**Adults 50-75**
High Blood Pressure Screening	**Adults 18+**
Tobacco Use Counseling	**Adults 18+**
Breast Cancer Mammogram	**Women 50-74**
Depression Screening	**Teens, Adults 18+**
Health Diet Counseling	**Adults with risk of heart disease**
Obesity Screening	**Children 6-17, Adults 18+**
Type 2 Diabetes Screening	**Adults with high blood pressure**

As for immunizations, those recommended by the Centers for Disease Control and Prevention will be deemed part of the "essential health benefits" package that all insurance plans must cover under the new law.

Employer-Based Personal Wellness Reward Programs

With approved preventive tests guaranteed to all Americans, ObamaCare also puts an emphasis on employer-based insurance plans to help improve the personal wellness of the population. Opening a new door for employers, the law permits them to offer financial rewards to their employees who make a measurable effort toward improving their health.

Specifically, it lets an employer reduce the premiums, co-pays and deductibles of its employees who meet specific personal wellness thresholds. Under the same conditions it also lets them increase the benefits employees can receive under a given insurance plan. As of 2011 the total value of the financial reward an employer can offer to an employee who meets a personal wellness standard is capped at 30 percent of the cost of the employee's total coverage. In 2014 employers may increase the reward level to 50 percent.

? DID YOU KNOW . . .

You won't only encounter ObamaCare when you go to see your doctor; as of 2011 all restaurants with 20 or more locations have to provide nutritional information and calorie counts on their menus.

To prevent employers from unfairly discriminating against less healthy workers, the law requires that they set up a different standard for employees who cannot reasonably meet those set up in the insurance plan for the employer's workforce as a whole.

A report reviewing the operation of employer-based wellness programs throughout the United States will be issued by 2013. In addition, small businesses will have access to grants to help them overcome any unique challenges they may have compared to larger businesses in setting up such programs. These grants will begin in 2011 and end in 2016.

Moving beyond employer-based plans, ObamaCare also sets up an extensive pilot program in 2014 whereby private insurance plans in 10 states will be encouraged to set up similar wellness programs. At the conclusion of three years, the pilot program will be reviewed and, if it proves effective, it could be expanded to more states in 2017

Nutritional Information in Restaurants

You won't only encounter ObamaCare when you go to see your doctor; its provisions will also affect you when you go to a restaurant. As of 2011 all restaurants with 20 or more locations have to provide nutritional information and calorie counts on their menus. Vending machines must do the same.

Increased Funding for Preventive Services in Medicaid

Under provisions that took effect in 2011, Medicaid now only covers preventive services approved by the U.S. Preventive Services Task Force. As with all other insurance plans, co-pays will be eliminated for those procedures that receive the task force's "A" or "B" rating. More importantly, states that provide Medicaid coverage for the recommended procedures and eliminate co-pays will receive a 1 percent increase in the so-called "federal medical assistance percentage" (or FMAP) for these services.

This aims to encourage states to support prevention efforts and Medicaid recipients themselves are given incentives to live healthier lives. Although specifics about these incentives remain vague, one initiative that was explicitly written into the new law requires Medicaid to cover tobacco-cessation services and products for pregnant women.

Prevention Counseling in Medicare

As with Medicaid, Medicare recipients are encouraged to live healthier lives, with a handful of new incentives, including the elimination of co-pays for approved preventive procedures. To further help with that effort, Medicare recipients are able to work with their doctors to develop a prevention plan customized to their specific needs.

Additional Costs for a Healthier America

The new initiatives designed to foster prevention and wellness are a step in the right direction, but it's an open question whether or not they will truly improve the general health of the American people.

Ironically, perhaps, ObamaCare could actually increase health and medical costs rather than reduce them. More preventive tests may bring more diagnosed health problems that require costly treatment that will raise healthcare spending above current levels.

Although we should all want to extend human life as much as possible, we should not be blind to the fact that a healthier, longer-living population will require more healthcare.

Still, the United States' standing on life expectancy in the world has become something of a national embarrassment, especially given the gigantic amount of money we spend on healthcare compared to other developed nations. Improving the diets and lifestyles of Americans (assuming they can be improved by government policy) is probably at least as important as fixing the healthcare system itself.

LONG-TERM CARE

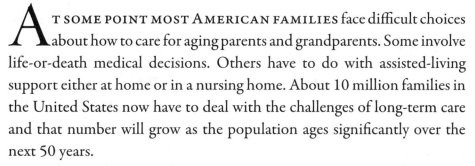

A T SOME POINT MOST AMERICAN FAMILIES face difficult choices about how to care for aging parents and grandparents. Some involve life-or-death medical decisions. Others have to do with assisted-living support either at home or in a nursing home. About 10 million families in the United States now have to deal with the challenges of long-term care and that number will grow as the population ages significantly over the next 50 years.

Realizing the growing importance of this issue and the financial burden it can impose on families, ObamaCare made an effort to help Americans care for old and/or disabled family members with new forms of government support, the most notable of which was the CLASS government run assisted-living insurance program. This aspect of the new law was the legacy of the late Senator Ted Kennedy, the foremost champion of a government-supported, long-term care program.

CLASS, however, was one of the most controversial parts of ObamaCare and the White House finally decided in October 2011 to pull the plug on it, admitting that the insurance plan could not sustain itself over the long term through enrollee contributions (participation in the plan was to be voluntary). This was a major victory for the legion of CLASS critics who had denounced the plan as another budget-busting entitlement and a major defeat for ObamaCare as CLASS was one of its most important components.

Although CLASS is now officially suspended, it has not been repealed by Congress. Because it could potentially come back to life in some form, we offer the following description of the plan as it stood before the White House's decision not to go forward with it.

CLASS Insurance

CLASS — short for "community living assistance services and supports" — was designed to be insurance that would provide financial help for those who cannot complete basic living tasks (such as feeding, dressing and bathing). People limited in this way are mostly senior citizens, but a sizeable portion of those who need such care (about 40 percent of the total) are under age 65 and disabled.

CLASS was intended to ease the heavy burden of assisted-living expenses for needy individuals and provide additional money so that they don't have to rely only on Medicaid, private insurance and their family's financial resources to make life bearable. It was not intended to cover all assisted-living expenses, but rather meant as a supplemental financial resource.

According to an insurance trade group, about 8 million long-term care policies exist in the United States today, with the average buyer in his or her late 50s and annual premiums a little over $2,000 per year. CLASS relied on these private policies as a general template to create the government's own insurance plan, the highlights of which are as follows:

- **Management and Oversight** — The CLASS program would be managed by the Department of Health and Human Services, which would determine the rules and set premium levels.

- **Voluntary Participation** — No one would be forced to contribute to CLASS. Any adult age 18 and older would be allowed to participate, either through their employer (if it offers CLASS as part of its insurance package) or directly through the government.

- **Payroll Deductions and Automatic Enrollment** — CLASS would be funded through payroll deductions, yet to be determined. Premiums would vary according to the age of the enrollee, with younger workers paying less than older ones. Importantly, health status cannot be used as a reason to charge higher premiums under CLASS. Employers who might offer CLASS to their workforce would have to automatically enroll each of their workers, but each enrollee would be able to opt out if they wish.

- **Start of Program** — The CLASS program was to have been created in 2011 with enrollments beginning in October 2012.

- **Five-Year Vesting Plan** — The plan would not pay out any benefits for the first five years of a person's enrollment. Enrollee contributions in the form of monthly premiums would build up slowly over time, eventually forming a self-sustaining pool of money to pay out benefits. The law specifies that CLASS must pay for itself and that taxpayer dollars may not be used to support payments to beneficiaries.

- **Benefit Eligibility** — All enrollees who have more than one functional limitation which impairs their ability to live a normal day-to-day life would be able to receive benefits. A doctor's certification would be required as proof that a limitation exists. To qualify for benefits, a person must have paid CLASS premiums for at least five years and have been employed for at least three of them.

- **Cash Benefit** — Many details of CLASS still need to be worked out, but the provision indicates those who qualify for benefits would receive a lifetime cash benefit amounting to, at minimum, $50 per day. The exact benefit level would be based on the severity of the functional limitation. If implemented, it's expected to amount to about $75 a day (or $27,375 per year) on average for all beneficiaries.

- **Use of Cash Benefit** — The money provided by CLASS could be used on pretty much anything that helps a person complete the daily tasks of life – including pay for an assistant in the home, housing modifications (e.g., making a bathroom accessible to a wheelchair) and transportation to shop for groceries. If a beneficiary resides in a nursing home, they may use CLASS money to pay those expenses.

- **Impact on Eligibility for Other Government Programs** — Participation in the CLASS program would not hinder a person's ability to receive Medicaid, Medicare, Social Security or any other government benefits. The program was designed to supplement these benefits, not replace them.

SO WHY DID THE WHITE HOUSE DECIDE NOT TO GO FORWARD WITH CLASS?
CLASS was deeply flawed because of its "opt out" provision. The Congressional Budget Office thought the non-participation level would be very high, with more than nine out of every 10 working adults ultimately opting out of CLASS.

Because CLASS benefits were guaranteed and because premiums could not be based on a person's health status, the largest number of enrollees would likely have been those who needed assisted-living care now or in the near future. Given these facts, CLASS was nothing less than an actuarial nightmare as the risk pool was almost guaranteed to be heavily lopsided toward the old and disabled, who by definition use more healthcare services than their payments cover.

In the short term, however, the CLASS program would have been smooth sailing from a budgetary standpoint. In its first five years it would have accumulated billions of dollars and it did not have to pay out any benefits at all during this time, thus making the ugly federal deficit look slightly better as government revenue increased on paper.

For many CLASS critics, the White House understood the plan was deeply flawed and insisted on including it in ObamaCare to create the revenues to fund the new law.

Over the next decade the CBO projected that CLASS would have taken in $70 billion in surplus revenue from an average monthly premium of $123. With that extra $70 billion created through budgetary sleight-of-hand the administration was able to claim that ObamaCare actually would reduce the federal budget deficit.

Despite White House reassurances, fears about CLASS were prevalent before ObamaCare's passage. "This is a scary proposition where the government passes a huge new entitlement program with gimmicks and tricks and the American people don't know they will be automatically enrolled in it by their employer if they don't watch out," said Devin Nunes, a Republican Congressman from California who opposed ObamaCare.

Even those who voted for ObamaCare had concerns about CLASS. Six Democrats in the Senate and Independent Senator Joe Lieberman refused to support it. Senator Kent Conrad, a Democrat from North Dakota, called CLASS a "Ponzi scheme" and "something that Bernie Madoff would be proud of."

He used that characterization because the money taken in over the first five years would not have been put in a designated government bank account, but would have been used instead to fund other federal programs. Like Social Security payments made to beneficiaries today, the only thing that would have funded CLASS when it came time to pay out benefits would have been paper IOU's, not real money. Fortunately, with the demise of CLASS these fears have disappeared.

Promoting In-Home, Long-Term Care

Medicaid is often thought of as the government program that provides healthcare for children and poor Americans. That perception is true enough, but about one-third of its budget (around $100 billion each year) also funds assisted-living and nursing home care, much of it for senior citizens. Medicare, the program we most think of as helping to care for seniors, does not provide such support.

? DID YOU KNOW . . .

Under ObamaCare, Medicaid will expand to help states provide assistance to those who live in their own homes, but need help living day-to-day – to encourage seniors to stay out of more expensive nursing homes.

Under ObamaCare, Medicaid will continue to provide long-term care as it has in the past for those who live in nursing homes. But the new law strives to broaden the reach of the program to include those who live in their own homes, who need help living day-to-day. It does this by offering states more federal money for in-home, assisted-living care, the net effect of which will be to encourage seniors to stay out of more expensive nursing homes.

In showering financial support on the nursing home industry over the years Medicaid has inadvertently undermined in-home and community-based, assisted-living services. Most seniors would understandably prefer to avoid being sent into a nursing home, where they are disconnected from their families. ObamaCare makes a sensible effort to align Medicaid with this preference.

The new law also loosens Medicaid eligibility rules as they apply to long-term care. In the past a married couple would have had to exhaust all savings and assets in order to qualify for Medicaid long-term care benefits.

Now, spouses will be able to retain more financial resources without hurting his or her partner's chances of receiving help through Medicaid.

Helping "Dual Eligibles"

One of the biggest challenges for anyone who needs long-term care is dealing with the government bureaucracy that is the gatekeeper to assisted-living benefits. For a senior citizen who has one or more chronic ailments and needs day-to-day assistance, that means getting help from both Medicare and Medicaid. In most cases, Medicare supports their medical needs, but Medicaid covers the rest of their non-medical care.

According to the Kaiser Foundation, almost 10 million people receive both Medicaid and Medicare benefits. These so-called "dual eligibles" are the most needy Americans receiving government assistance. More than $200 billion is spent each year to care for them and, on a per-capita basis, they require four times as much spending as "non-duals." And yet, despite the financial burden generated by this group, very little attention has been paid to them.

ObamaCare seeks to change that. For the first time Medicare and Medicaid will be encouraged to work together much more than they have in the past in delivering services to "dual eligibles." The Department of Health and Human Services will create a new "Federal Coordinated Healthcare Office," which will coordinate the delivery of benefits to this important group. The new office will streamline bureaucratic procedures for "dual eligibles," remove regulatory conflicts between Medicare and Medicaid and eliminate any unnecessary overlap in care.

Nursing Home Transparency and Improvement

Medicaid enhancements are largely focused on helping provide better long-term care for people who stay in their own homes, but ObamaCare also tries to improve the condition of those who reside in nursing homes.

Under the law, nursing homes must comply with an array of new rules and regulations intended to protect the elderly who live in such facilities and improve the quality of their lives. Here are the highlights:

- **Ownership Disclosure** — In recent years many nursing homes have been bought by private investment firms, attracted to the business because of the stable revenue streams generated by Medicare and Medicaid. This trend has made it more difficult to pinpoint the parties accountable when the level of care falls to an unacceptable level. The new law requires ownership transparency of all nursing homes so that the voices of residents are not ignored.

- **State Monitoring** — Each state will be required to gather information on the performance of nursing homes and provide public access to this information on a website. They must also make available a standardized complaint form that residents and their families can use to take action against a specific nursing home.

- **Metrics on Nursing Home Quality** — Each facility will be required to reveal information about the size and quality of its staff, how much they're paid, the hours of care they provide to residents each day, their turnover and retention rates, the number and type of complaints against them, and their criminal records if they have them. Nursing homes will also be required to reveal any penalties that their facilities have received in the past.

- **Website Tool** — Newly collected information about nursing home performance and quality will be provided on the *Medicare.gov* website in conjunction with its "Nursing Home Compare" tool.

- **Ethics Programs** — To help reduce poor care and criminal activity, each facility will establish rules of conduct for its staff and publicly reveal levels of compliance.

- **Notice of Closure** — All nursing homes will be required to give at least 60 days notice to residents if they intend to close.

WHAT ABOUT "DEATH PANELS"?

A big controversy in the national debate over ObamaCare came when Sarah Palin posted the following statement on her Facebook page: "The America I know and love is not one in which my parents or my baby with Down syndrome will have to stand in front of Obama's 'death panel' so his bureaucrats can decide, based on a subjective judgment of their 'level of productivity in society,' whether they are worthy of healthcare. Such a system is downright evil."

Palin's fears were fueled by a provision written into the health reform legislation by Democrats in the House of Representatives that funded voluntary consultations between doctors and Medicare recipients about end-of-life issues, touching on such things as living wills and hospice care.

She was also disturbed by the controversial views of one of President Obama's advisers on healthcare reform, Dr. Ezekiel Emanuel, the brother of former White House Chief of Staff, Rahm Emanuel. Palin was reacting in part to Dr. Emanuel's controversial statements about end-of-life care in which he pointed out that as much as 80 percent of a person's healthcare costs come at the end of their life and that "some independent group that can give you advice" was required to help reduce such expenditures.

If you remember this controversy and worry that you or a member of your family will one day have to deal with a "death panel," there is reason not to worry.

ObamaCare guarantees that the government must "ensure that the health benefits established as essential not be subject to denial to individuals against their wishes on the basis of the individual's age or expected length of life or the individual's present or predicted disability, degree of medical dependency or quality of life."

A sticky point is that the phrase "essential health benefits" has not yet been defined by the Obama Administration. A general outline of the essential health benefits was announced in November 2012, but no specific information about coverage was included (see Appendix A).

OBAMACARE, ETC. 14

ObamaCare calls for a series of sweeping changes in certain segments of the healthcare industry that will have a ripple effect on everything from how insurance companies will cover people who retire from the workforce before age 65 to the regulation of physican-owned hospitals, the way doctors currently do business, and the operation of federally funded community health centers that serve needy populations.

Early Retiree Reinsurance Plan

With so much of ObamaCare devoted to decreasing the uninsured population, many of whom are in early adulthood, it's easy to forget that the new law also includes a provision that helps those at the other end of the age spectrum who have recently left the nation's labor force.

Specifically, it calls for a new reinsurance program that encourages employers to continue to provide health insurance to their early retirees over the age of 55 but younger than 65 (the age the retirees become eligible for Medicare). Under the reinsurance plan the federal government reimburses employers for 80 percent of insurance claims between $15,000 and $90,000. The program began in mid-2010 with $5 billion in federal financing behind it and will be discontinued in January 2014. At that point early retirees will be able to buy health insurance through state-based exchanges.

By the end of 2010 almost 4,000 employers and unions had signed up for the reinsurance program. Unlike the government's "high-risk pool" for individuals who cannot get coverage because they have a pre-existing health condition, the retiree reinsurance program is off to a good start.

Restrictions on Physician-Owned Hospitals

It's not an exaggeration to say that ObamaCare declares war on physician-owned hospitals. There is no official ban on these institutions (those that exist now can still operate), but new ones constructed after December 31, 2010, will no longer be certified by Medicare, and thus will not be able to access this all-important revenue stream, which most hospitals need to survive. Exemptions are possible under some circumstances, so some physician-owned hospitals could still be built. But their growth will be seriously curtailed by the new law.

ObamaCare's war on physician-owned hospitals comes in response to criticism of these institutions made by community and non-profit hospitals, which have argued that they focus on lucrative specialties such as orthopedics and cardiac care and push money-losing efforts such as emergency room care onto them.

However valid this criticism may be, the restriction on physician-owned hospitals is ill-timed. More than 30 million more Americans will have to obtain health insurance because of ObamaCare's individual mandate and as a consequence the demand for services will steadily increase over the next decade. When it does, a bottleneck could form in the healthcare system, making it more difficult to obtain care. The United

States will need more hospitals, even those that do not provide a broad level of community care.

Help could be on the way to lift the restriction. By the end of 2010 lawsuits on behalf of doctor-owned hospitals had already been filed in federal court, with the Physicians Hospitals of America, a lobbying group, arguing that the new law restricting doctor-owned hospitals is "retroactive, arbitrary, vague, contradictory, and violates due process and equal protection." Time will tell whether or not this argument proves persuasive.

Doctor Shortages Forecast

Critics of ObamaCare assert that the new law will decrease both the quality and number of American doctors, and do so at a time when their services will be in higher demand than ever before. If their prediction comes true, the consequences for healthcare in the United States would be disastrous. Not only would it become much harder to find a doctor, the price you would have to pay for their services could rise significantly.

> **❓ DID YOU KNOW . . .**
>
> The Association of American Medical Colleges estimates that by 2015 the country will need 60,000 more doctors than it is expected to have by then. It expects the shortage to worsen through 2025.

Will this doomsday scenario actually happen? As with so much of the law's future impact, it's hard to say. A growing consensus, however, sees the potential for destabilization of the medical profession and a possible exodus as an unintended consequence of ObamaCare. The Association of American Medical Colleges, for instance, estimates that by 2015 the country will need 60,000 more doctors than it is expected to have by then. It expects the shortage to worsen through 2025.

Investors Business Daily predicts a much worse doctor shortage. By its estimate as many as 360,000 physicians could leave the profession rather than accept the changes that are coming. The newspaper's August 2009 forecast was based on a survey conducted among 1,300 doctors during the national debate over the new law.

The survey revealed significant dissatisfaction among the nation's physicians regarding the reform package that was ultimately pushed through Congress. Of those doctors who responded, 44 percent said that they "would consider leaving their practice or taking an early retirement" if Congress passed ObamaCare.

Some have suggested the timing of the poll — it was conducted right at the height of national debate on ObamaCare – dramatically inflated those numbers. Critics of the poll suggested the notion that more than 4 in 10 of the nation's doctors would choose a new career or simply stop practicing medicine rather than live by the new laws was simply preposterous.

❓ DID YOU KNOW . . .

ObamaCare provides $11 billion in funding for community health centers, which are federal subsidized clinics that provide healthcare for uninsured Americans in underserved areas such as inner cities and rural locales.

Supporters of the new law attacked the *Investors Business Daily* survey, branding it a partisan distortion with no merit, but it was more or less confirmed by a more recent survey of 2,400 doctors. Commissioned by the Physicians Foundation, the new poll was conducted at the end of 2010. As with the previous poll, a large number of the doctors surveyed (40 percent) expressed dissatisfaction, claiming that they would "retire, seek a non-clinical job in healthcare, or seek a job or business unrelated to healthcare" before the big pieces of ObamaCare are implemented in 2014.

While it's unlikely that four out of every 10 doctors will actually leave their profession because of ObamaCare (survey claims about future behavior rarely match reality), some departures might occur. If even one in 10 doctors decides they don't want to participate in the new system, it will be a blow to the quality and availability of healthcare in the United States.

Funding for Community Health Centers

ObamaCare provides $11 billion in funding for community health centers, which are federal subsidized clinics that provide healthcare for uninsured Americans in underserved areas such as inner cities and rural locales.

The funding is recognition that despite the individual mandate, the expansion of Medicaid and the new healthcare exchanges, millions of people in the country will remain without insurance. The estimated 13 million illegal aliens, for example, will by law remain outside the system, but still need care. Community health centers will help address this problem and hospital emergency rooms will remain places where anyone without insurance can turn to receive care.

PART V

Crunching the Numbers

> " The truth is no one really knows how much ObamaCare costs since the actual price will hinge on behavior that can't be predicted. "

OBAMACARE'S PRICE TAG 15

OBAMACARE — THE MOST EXPENSIVE entitlement program created in the United States since Medicaid and Medicare were created almost 50 years ago — comes with a massive price tag of $1 trillion over the next decade. In an ordinary time of peace and prosperity that might be a number the American people could easily swallow, but these are not ordinary times.

As the United States continues to fight a prolonged, low-intensity war against radical Islamic terrorists, it is simultaneously burdened by an almost incomprehensible national debt of $14 trillion and growing. Viewed against this mountain of money, another trillion dollars thrown onto the pile might not seem like much of an additional burden. On the other hand, it might just be the straw that breaks the nation's back, especially if the real price of ObamaCare is significantly higher than what it's projected to cost by today's budget forecasters.

The authors of ObamaCare, knowing that the gigantic price of major healthcare reform could derail their efforts to make it a reality, took extra pains to finance the new healthcare system without adding to the nation's annual budget deficit. And according to the Congressional Budget Office

? DID YOU KNOW . . .

If the government's financial projections are accurate, new revenue-generating schemes will raise $1.2 trillion between 2010 and 2019 and be more than enough to cover the anticipated cost of ObamaCare over that time period.

they were successful, achieving significant reform that should, in theory, pay for itself without increasing the nation's debt.

President Obama and Congressional Democrats achieved this difficult-to-believe budgetary miracle by cutting the spending of existing programs such as Medicare and creating a whole new array of taxes, fees and penalties that the American people, employers and the healthcare industry as a whole will have to pay.

If the government's financial projections are accurate, these new revenue-generating schemes will raise $1.2 trillion between 2010 and 2019 and be more than enough to cover the anticipated cost of ObamaCare over that time period.

TAB. 15-1: OBAMACARE'S BUDGET (2010-2019, IN BILLIONS OF $)	
Revenue Generated By ObamaCare	$1,218
Cost of ObamaCare	$1,075
Applied To Deficit	$143

Source: Congressional Budget Office

NOTE ON CONGRESSIONAL BUDGET OFFICE OBAMACARE BUDGET FORECAST

The above numbers and those given in this book reflect the Congressional Budget Office's original estimate of the cost of ObamaCare. Since then the Supreme Court has ruled that states may opt out of the expansion of Medicaid, with the result that the government may have to pay for Medicaid coverage for millions fewer than it expected. It is impossible to say right now how many states will opt out, but the CBO believes the cost savings will be about $84 billion — a negligible amount given the law's $1 trillion price tag.

Amazing as it may sound, ObamaCare will not only pay for itself according to these official non-partisan projections, but will generate extra revenue to the tune of $143 billion, which in turn will be used to reduce the federal budget deficit. Citing these numbers, supporters of the new law were able to tell the American people that the large entitlement program they wanted to create would actually make the nation's financial condition better, not worse.

Should we believe the projection used to make this assertion? If history is any guide, the answer is no.

When we look at the original budget forecasts for other large entitlement programs like Social Security, Medicare and Medicaid, we see tremendous understatement of the actual long-term costs of these programs. Back in the 1960s, for instance, the House Ways and Means Committee (there was no Congressional Budget Office back then) predicted Medicare would cost $12 billion by 1990. The real number was almost $100 billion — more than eight times higher than the forecast.

❓ DID YOU KNOW . . .

ObamaCare will impose significant new fees on the pharmaceutical and health insurance industries that will generate $107 billion over the next decade, according to the Congressional Budget Office.

Families USA, a group that supported ObamaCare, commissioned an independent analysis of the CBO's forecast for the new healthcare system and discovered that it was wildly understated, particularly the estimate for the amount of money needed to provide subsidies on the health insurance exchanges. According to its analysis the actual amount needed to fund the exchanges in their first year (2014) will be more than five times higher than the CBO estimate.

One expert says one thing about the cost of ObamaCare and one says another. Whom should we believe? The answer is neither. All budget forecasters base their projections on assumptions that, in reality, are best guesses. The truth is no one really knows how much ObamaCare costs since the actual price will hinge on behavior that can't be predicted.

On the other hand, as Bob Dylan once said, you don't need a weather vane to know which way the wind is blowing. Common sense says that insuring more than 30 million people and simultaneously guaranteeing that every citizen has a plethora of new healthcare benefits will impose a significant financial burden on taxpayers that did not exist before ObamaCare's passage.

Where Does the Money Generated by ObamaCare Go?

If we want to boil ObamaCare down to its most important parts, all we need to do is look at what eats up most of its budget.

Two big pieces of the new healthcare system immediately jump off ObamaCare's balance sheet — the expansion of Medicaid and the health insurance exchanges. Taken together, they constitute an overwhelming 84 percent of the cost of the new law or about $900 billion, with the exchanges costing $465 billion and the expansion of Medicaid costing another $434 billion. The rest of ObamaCare's spending ($176 billion) is window dressing in comparison.

TAB. 15-2: **THE PRICE OF OBAMACARE (2010-2019, BILLIONS OF $)**		
Total Cost Of ObamaCare	**$1,075**	100.0%
Health Insurance Exchanges	**$465**	**43.3%**
Premium and Co-Pay Subsidies	$350	32.6%
Exchange Premium Credits	$107	10.0%
Startup Costs/Other	$8	0.7%
Medicaid Expansion/CHIP	**$434**	**40.4%**
All Other Costs	**$176**	**16.4%**
Reinsurance & Risk Adjustment	$106	9.9%
Small Employer Tax Credits	$37	3.4%
Other	$33	3.1%

Where Does the Money for ObamaCare Come From?

In order to pay for ObamaCare over the next decade, President Obama and Congressional Democrats cobbled together revenue from a variety of sources, but one stands out prominently: Medicare. The largest source of funding for the new healthcare system comes from Medicare spending cuts, followed by an assortment of new taxes and fees imposed across the board. Let's take a closer look at each revenue source.

TAB. 15-3: **REVENUE GENERATED BY OBAMACARE (2010-2019, BILLIONS OF $)**		
Total Revenue For ObamaCare	$1,218*	100.0%
Medicare Spending Cuts	$455	37.4%
Medicare Payment Rate Cuts	$196	16.1%
Medicare Advantage Cuts	$136	11.2%
Other Medicare/Medicaid Cuts	$123	10.1%
New Taxes And Fees	$414	34.0%
Hospital Insurance/Unearned Income Tax	$210	17.2%
Fees on Insurers & Drug Companies	$107	8.8%
Individual & Employer Penalty	$65	5.3%
Excise Tax On "Cadillac" Plans	$32	2.6%
All Other Revenue Sources	$349	28.7%
Other Revenue Provisions	$108	8.9%
Reinsurance & Risk Adjustment	$106	8.7%
Community Assisted Living	$70	5.7%
Positive Effects On Revenue	$46	3.8%
Education Cuts	$19	1.6%

Source:*$143 billion of this applied to federal budget deficit, $1,075 to fund ObamaCare

Medicare Spending Cuts

The ObamaCare cuts to Medicare's budget are discussed at length in another section of this book, chapter 10 entitled, "Turning the Screws on Medicare."

Increased Medicare Hospital Insurance Tax

One of the biggest sources of revenue for ObamaCare besides Medicare spending cuts will come in the form of an increase in the Medicare hospital insurance tax that American workers pay. The current tax is 2.90 percent, with the employer and employee both contributing 1.45 percent. The new law raises the employee portion of this tax to 2.35 percent for high-income earners, specifically for individuals who make more than $200,000 per year and for couples who make more than $250,000 per year. After the increase goes into effect in 2013, the new hospital insurance tax (employer and employee's share combined) will be 3.80 percent on income above the new thresholds.

TAB. 15-4: **INCREASED MEDICARE HOSPITAL INSURANCE TAX (2013 & AFTER)**			
	Income	**Before ObamaCare**	**After ObamaCare**
Individuals	< $200K	1.45%	1.45%
	> $200K	1.45%	2.35%
Families	< $250K	1.45%	1.45%
	> $250K	1.45%	2.35%

Increased Medicare Unearned Income/Investment Tax

Another important source of revenue will come from the Medicare contribution tax imposed on individuals making more than $200,000 per year and couples earning at least $250,000 per year. The tax will only apply to investment income (such as capital gains, interest, dividends, annuities, royalties and rents) above the income thresholds. The new tax will go into effect January 1, 2013.

TAB. 15-5: **NEW MEDICARE INVESTMENT INCOME TAX (2013 & AFTER)**			
	Income	Before ObamaCare	After ObamaCare
Individuals	>$200K	0%	0%
	> $200K	0%	3.80%
Families	< $250K	0%	0%
	> $250K	0%	3.80%

This new 3.8 percent tax has raised fears that it represents a new "transfer tax" on the capital gains of homeowners when they realize a profit from the sale of their home. While in some cases the tax could apply to home sales in this way, most Americans will not be affected by it. Here's why:

- Some may be wondering, what if they sell their house for a big profit and vault over the $250,000 threshold in a given year? Won't they have to pay the tax then? Probably not if they live in the home they are selling. In the 1990s, President Clinton signed into law an exemption to the capital gains tax for those who sell their own home and realize a profit under $500,000 (married couples) and $250,000 (individuals). Clinton's exemption is still in place and the new ObamaCare 3.8 percent surtax only applies above the $500,000 and $250,000 profit levels.

- Right now, a married couple that realizes a capital gains profit exceeding $500,000 on the sale of a home must pay a 15 percent tax on the amount above this level. The ObamaCare surtax of 3.8 percent raises it to 18.8 percent

- For those who are selling homes they don't live in, the 3.8 percent tax will apply to capital gains above the ObamaCare thresholds since these individuals will not enjoy the benefit of Clinton's exemption.

Taken together, the two new Medicare taxes imposed on high-income earners (the hospital insurance tax and the investment income tax) are expected to generate $210 billion in revenue over the next decade or about 17 percent of the funding needed to pay for ObamaCare.

New Fees on Pharmaceutical and Health Insurance Industries

ObamaCare will impose significant new fees on the pharmaceutical and health insurance industries that will generate $107 billion over the next decade, according to the Congressional Budget Office. The fees will be phased in over time as shown for the healthcare industry in Table 15-6. Pharmaceutical industry fees (not shown) will gradually increase in the same way.

TAB. 15-6: **NEW ANNUAL FEES ON HEALTH INSURANCE INDUSTRY (BILLIONS $)**		
Year	Before ObamaCare	After ObamaCare
2014	None	$8.0
2015	None	$11.3
2016	None	$11.3
2017	None	$13.9
2018	None	$11.3

*Amount for each year after pegged to rise in premium costs

The new fees on these industries are expected to generate about 9 percent of ObamaCare's revenue over the next decade. The affected industries have accepted these fees without protest largely because of the 30 million additional customers that ObamaCare pushes onto their doorstep with money in hand ready to buy health insurance and prescription drugs. By their calculation, financial gains from this bigger market will more than offset the $107 billion they have agreed to pay the government.

Financial Penalties on Individuals and Employers

The fines imposed on Americans who do not get health insurance and a similar penalty imposed on employers who do not offer coverage to their employees are primarily intended to decrease the number of uninsured in the United States.

But they will also generate significant revenue that helps fund ObamaCare because some people and businesses will not comply. In aggregate, the amount generated by the penalties is expected to reach $65 billion over the next decade or about 5 percent of ObamaCare's revenue. But opponents of the individual mandate who say that it was put in place to pay for ObamaCare paint a distorted picture as nearly all of the new healthcare system's funding (95 percent) will come from other sources.

Excise Tax on "Cadillac" Health Insurance Plans

Hoping to simultaneously generate revenue and discourage excessive spending on healthcare by Americans (the authors of the new law are convinced that "overutilization" raises costs for everyone), ObamaCare imposes a heavy 40 percent tax on "Cadillac" insurance plans.

Despite what the label "Cadillac" implies, expensive health insurance plans are held by a broader range of people than Wall Street tycoons and wealthy industrialists. The higher price paid for them is often a function of the holder's age and health status, not his or her net financial worth. Many union workers, for instance, have plans that fall into the "Cadillac" category, and this is one reason unions opposed the tax (see Appendix A).

Although the tax is imposed on the insurer, not the policyholder, that is probably a distinction without a difference since it is likely to be passed on to the customer, raising the overall price of the insurance plan and the premiums associated with it. Showing the power of interest groups opposed

> **? DID YOU KNOW . . .**
> Beginning in 2013 employers will only be able to make tax-free contributions to an employee's flexible savings account up to $2,500 per year.

to it, the new tax won't take effect until 2018. No one really knows for sure whether the tax will actually be imposed when the time comes.

	Plan Value	Before ObamaCare	After ObamaCare
TAB. 15-7: **EXCISE TAX ON "CADILLAC" HEALTHCARE PLANS (2018 & AFTER)**			
Individuals	< $10,200	0%	0%
	> $10,200	0%	40%*
Families	< $27,500	0%	0%
	> $27,500	0%	40%

*Tax imposed on amount above plan value on the insurer who issues it

How will the new tax work exactly? Health insurance plans in 2018 and the years after that which exceed $10,200 in premiums for an individual or $27,500 in premiums for a family (excluding dental and vision coverage) will be taxed at a rate of 40 percent above the threshold. While these thresholds may seem very high today, keep in mind they are not adjusted upward for inflation.

The Congressional Budget Office expects that the "Cadillac" plan tax will generate $32 billion or about 3 percent of ObamaCare's funding during its limited two years of operation within the law's current budget, with $12 billion raised in 2018 and $19 billion raised in 2019, respectively.

If, hypothetically speaking, this tax had been imposed in 2011 and generated a commensurate level of revenue each year, it would have raised $150 billion or more for ObamaCare over a decade. Assuming ObamaCare survives into the 2020s, the tax on "Cadillac" plans is likely to become one of the new healthcare system's biggest revenue sources.

Beginning in 2012 employers will be required for the first time to list the value of the health insurance they provide on employees' IRS W-2 forms documenting their earnings for the year. It's one small step from there to slap a new tax on healthcare benefits that have already been given income equivalency on paper by the government.

On a positive note, having Americans see the price of their health insurance revealed with a specific number could be a good thing. Few people realize how much their coverage costs as employers usually don't share this information with their workers. Many experts believe overuse of the healthcare system is one of the biggest factors driving up costs and comes in part because many Americans don't pay directly for most of their healthcare. Attaching a hard number to the value of their benefits might help change this behavior for the better.

Many Americans might be surprised to discover that, on average, employers pay about $13,500 per employee for health insurance, and that employees only pay about 30 percent – $4,000, on average – of the total amount in any given year. That's $333 a month per employee.

Higher Penalty for Health Savings Account Disbursement

To help fund the new healthcare system, ObamaCare increases the tax penalty from 10 to 20 percent for non-allowable purchases made using tax deductible funds in Health Savings Accounts (HSAs) and Flexible Spending Accounts (FSAs).

The Congressional Budget Office expects this provision to generate a modest $1.4 billion to help fund ObamaCare, leading some critics of the law to assert that this provision has more to do with limiting the freedom of Americans to make their own healthcare choices than with funding the new healthcare system. That argument has some merit because, as of 2011, HSA and FSA funds may only be used to buy prescription drugs, whereas in the past they could be used to buy over-the-counter drugs as well.

In other words, when someone who has one of these accounts goes to buy Advil or Tylenol, he or she will need to get a prescription from the doctor first in order to use tax-free funds. Many won't bother as the visit to their doctor will cost them more in time and money than the amount they would save if they had a prescription in hand.

TAB. 15-8: **CHANGES TO HEALTH SAVINGS ACCOUNTS (2011 & AFTER)**		
	Before ObamaCare	**After ObamaCare**
Tax Penalty For Non-Allowable Disbursements	10%	20%
Can Use To Buy OTC Drugs?	Yes	No

The critics predict that this new tax provision will lead to more prescriptions written for over-the-counter drugs by doctors. They fear that it will also spur sales of prescription drugs, even when a cheaper over-the-counter alternative will do. If this happens, consumer spending on drugs could increase because of the new law.

New Limits for Flexible Spending Accounts

Beginning in 2013 employers will only be able to make tax-free contributions to an employee's flexible savings account up to $2,500 per year, whereas the amount they could contribute in the past was unlimited.

The Congressional Budget Office expects this provision of the new law to generate $13 billion in funding for ObamaCare over the next decade. But more importantly it represents (like the new tax on "Cadillac" insurance plans) a restriction placed on employer-provided healthcare benefits and as such is more evidence supporting the case that ObamaCare may undermine today's employer-based health insurance system.

TAB. 15-9: **CHANGES TO FLEXIBLE SPENDING ACCOUNTS (2013 & AFTER)**		
	Before ObamaCare	**After ObamaCare**
Amount Employers Can Contribute To Employee's FSA Tax Free	Unlimited	Up To $2,500 Per Year

Excise Tax on Medical Devices

Starting in 2012 ObamaCare imposes a 2.3 percent excise tax on the manufacturer or importer of medical devices. Some devices are excluded, including glasses, contact lens, hearing aids and other devices available for retail purchase. The new tax is expected to raise $20 billion over the next decade.

TAB. 15-10: **EXCISE TAX ON MEDICAL DEVICES (2012 & AFTER)**		
	Before ObamaCare	**After ObamaCare**
Tax on Sale of Medical Devices	0%	2.3%

Medical Expenses Deduction Threshold Raised

Today Americans can deduct medical expenses that exceed 7.5 percent of their income from their taxes. That level increases to 10 percent under ObamaCare. This provision of the new law takes effect in 2013, but will not be extended to senior citizens until 2017. It's expected to generate about $15 billion over the next decade since fewer Americans will have expenses that exceed the 10 percent threshold.

TAB. 15-11: **TAX DEDUCTION FOR MEDICAL EXPENSES (2013 & AFTER)**		
	Before ObamaCare	**After ObamaCare**
Threshold Before Income Tax Deduction On Medical Expenses Can Be Claimed	7.5% of Income	10.0% of Income*

*Will apply to those age 65 and over beginning in 2017

Tax on Tanning Salons

In order to simultaneously discourage unhealthy practices and raise revenue for the new healthcare system, ObamaCare imposes a new 10 percent tax on indoor tanning services, which must be paid either by the tanning salon or the customer. This new tax is expected to raise about $3 billion in revenue over the next decade.

TAB. 15-12: **TAX ON INDOOR TANNING (2010 & AFTER)**		
	Before ObamaCare	**After ObamaCare**
Tax on Amount Paid for Indoor Tanning Services	0%	10%

CLASS Funds Counted as Revenue

Although a further $70 billion is counted as revenue to fund ObamaCare in the government's budgetary calculations, this money actually was projected to come from enrollee contributions into the now discontinued CLASS long-term care insurance plan. In other words, it was not free and clear revenue at all, but money that would have eventually been needed to pay beneficiaries.

This budgetary legerdemain might seem of minor importance, but it highlights the reality that the government's financial claims are not always what they seem to be at first glance. If we subtract this $70 billion from ObamaCare's revenue total (as we should since CLASS has been officially suspended), the real amount devoted to reducing the budget deficit is $73 billion and not $143 billion.

PART VI

LOOKING AHEAD

To paraphrase Bette Davis's famous advice in the movie *All About Eve*: "Buckle your seat belts. It's going to be a bumpy ride."

PROTECT YOURSELF AGAINST OBAMACARE | 16

Now that we've gone through ObamaCare piece by piece, you might be wondering what you can do to protect yourself from potential downsides of the new law and, on the flip side, how you might benefit from it. Here are a few suggestions:

Check Your Eligibility for Medicaid

If you're living on a low income, the dramatic expansion of Medicaid under ObamaCare could very well help you. At the very least, you should check to see if you are now eligible for the program. As we've discussed, a handful of states could refuse to loosen their eligibility requirements to enroll in Medicaid.

If you happen to live in one of these states, the future is uncertain. You will probably receive financial assistance, but it may not be enough to make your coverage free.

If you are in one of the 40 or more states that will expand their Medicaid enrollment in 2014, then you might be able to sign up for the program at that time. Under the new law every American who earns less

GOOD ADVICE:

If you make the determination not to get health insurance, the new law says you will have to pay a fine. Should you pay it? All of us should comply with the law, but having said this, it will probably be wise to see to what extent the fine is enforced before you write your check to the IRS.

than 133 percent of the federal poverty level (that's $29,327 for a family of four in 2010) will be able to enroll.

On the downside, if you live in a state like Minnesota that currently lets people into Medicaid above the 133 percent threshold, you might lose your eligibility. If you are currently in the program with an income above this level, you will in all likelihood be transferred to the health insurance exchange in your state, where you will receive a generous subsidy to help defray the cost of your coverage. This is a good deal, but not as good as Medicaid, which pays all of the cost. On the other hand, the private plan that you enroll in via the exchange may be more widely accepted than Medicaid by doctors and providers.

Don't Pay the Individual Mandate Penalty Unless You Have To

Now that the individual mandate has been ruled constitutional by the Supreme Court, it is likely to be a part of our lives.

But before you lose sleep about the financial penalty that it promises to impose on you if you don't obtain health insurance, you should first consider your own health insurance situation. If you have coverage (and 84 percent of Americans currently do), you won't have to pay any penalty because you comply with the law by that fact.

If you are among the much smaller group of Americans who don't have health insurance (16 percent of the population, including illegal aliens), you could still be eligible for Medicaid or subsidized coverage through your state's insurance exchange. Either alternative (where you will have to pay relatively little out of your own pocket, if anything at all) is likely to be a better option than paying the penalty.

After all, when you buy health insurance, at least you get something for your money. When you pay the ObamaCare penalty you get nothing in return.

If you make the determination not to get health insurance, the new law says you will have to pay a fine. Should you pay it? All of us should comply with the law, but having said this, it will probably be wise to see to what extent the fine is enforced before you write your check to the IRS. Because of the political firestorm swirling around the individual mandate, it might not be enforced at all.

Keep in mind that the law empowers the Internal Revenue Service to confiscate individual tax refunds to force you to pay money you owe the government. It still remains to be seen whether or not Congress will actually fund this effort, however, as it will require paying the salaries of thousands of new Internal Revenue Service agents who have yet to be hired.

! GOOD ADVICE:
You should check with your employer to see if it has set up a personal wellness reward program.

Get OTC Prescriptions if You Use a Health Savings Account

As of 2011, Americans who use Health Savings Accounts (HSAs) or Flexible Spending Accounts (FSAs) are no longer able to dip into these tax-free funds to pay for over-the-counter drugs like Tylenol and Tagamet. Under the new law, a doctor's prescription will be required for all OTC drug purchases in order to use HSA or FSA money to pay for them.

So, if you use a HSA or FSA and know that you will require certain OTC drugs in the future (for example, the OTC version of Claritin for your chronic allergy condition), you should try to get a prescription from your doctor in anticipation of your eventual need.

Get Approved Preventive Tests Without Being Charged Co-Pays

ObamaCare requires all insurance plans to cover so-called "essential health benefits" and among these are preventive tests that the government's task force on prevention has given an "A" or "B" certification.

Visit the task force's website at ***http://epss.ahrq.gov*** (the Agency for Healthcare Research and Quality) to see whether the preventive test you need is recommended. If it is, your insurance plan must pay for it without charging you a co-pay.

Therefore, if you feel the need for an approved test, you should get it as it will cost you nothing. This assumes, of course, that your employer's plan has not been granted "grandfathered" status. If it has, the new rule will not apply.

Check to See if Your Employer Has a Personal Wellness Reward Program

Under ObamaCare employers will be able to set up personal wellness reward programs within the insurance plans that they offer to their employees. If your employer has begun to use a wellness program, it could mean that you will have to pay higher premiums and co-pays than your co-workers if you don't meet the personal wellness standards established within your plan.

You should check with your employer to see if it has set up a personal wellness reward program. If it has, you should think about how easily you'll be able to meet the wellness standard in the plan. If you believe you may not be able to meet it, you should ask for a special exemption that allows you to opt out of the program. Otherwise, you could end up paying premiums and co-pays that are up to 50 percent higher than your peers.

Use the Government's "High-Risk" Insurance Pool if You Need To

Although ObamaCare required all insurance companies in September 2010 to cover children even if they had a pre-existing health condition, the same rule does not go into effect for adults until January 2014. If in the meantime you're not able to obtain health insurance because you have a pre-existing health condition, you have an alternative. The government has created a temporary "high-risk" insurance pool to help Americans in your situation between now and 2014.

This is your best bet to obtain coverage during this timeframe and now is a good time to sign up. Enrollment in the high-risk pool has gotten off to a slow start, with relatively few people joining the program by the end of 2010. Premiums have been lowered as a result.

If You're an Early Retiree Under Age 65, Prepare to Lose Your Insurance in 2014

With the creation of the state-based exchanges in 2014 many companies are expected to drop the insurance they provide to their early retirees under the age of 65. One big company, 3M, has already announced that it will do this because lower cost options will arrive with the exchanges. Once these are up and running, you will probably need to use them to buy your health insurance.

Medicare Advantage Enrollees Might Need to Find an Alternative

Given ObamaCare's reduction of the Medicare Advantage budget over the next decade, some insurers may decide to drop out of the program. If this happens, enrollees will have to look elsewhere for supplemental coverage to their basic Medicare benefits. You should plan for this possibility if you currently are part of Medicare Advantage.

If You're a High Earner, Talk to Your Accountant

High earners are specifically targeted by ObamaCare as a revenue source to fund the new healthcare system. The money will be generated by new Medicare contribution taxes relating to hospital insurance and investment income, with individuals who make more than $200,000 per year and couples who earn at least $250,000 having to pay more than in the past.

❗ GOOD ADVICE:

You can continue to get the latest updates on the ObamaCare law and its impact on you by signing up for a free email alert by going to *www. SurvivingObamaCare.com.*

Although it will be difficult to avoid these new taxes if you fall into this group, you should nonetheless talk with your accountant to determine the best approach to dealing with them, assuming there is a best approach.

Small Business Owners Should Calculate Health-related Costs of New Hires

Because ObamaCare gives a substantial tax credit to small businesses that employ 25 or fewer people, the owners of these enterprises should think carefully about whether or not they should expand their workforce. The full tax credit is available for those businesses with 10 or fewer workers so there is now less incentive to hire more than 10 employees than there was in past.

Whether or not such a decision makes financial sense for your business is a calculation you will have to make on your own. If a significant number of small businesses choose to limit their employees because they are incentivized by the tax credit to do so, the nation's overall employment outlook could be hurt, and if it is, ObamaCare will generate another unwelcome, unintended consequence.

Stay Informed

Under our system of government, laws aren't written in stone. Congress can modify or repeal them; the president can refuse to enforce them; and the courts can strike them down and election results can change both the nature and implementation of laws. Like any other law in the initial period after its enactment, ObamaCare lives in a fluid state. It's likely that new developments will cause the law to mutate into something different from what it is today.

You can continue to get the latest updates on the ObamaCare law and its impact on you by signing up for a free email alert by going to *www.SurvivingObamaCare.com*.

This book paints a picture of ObamaCare in the middle of 2012. You will need to pay attention to the news in the days ahead to take note of important changes as they come along.

To paraphrase Bette Davis's famous advice in the movie *All About Eve*: "Buckle your seat belts. It's going to be a bumpy ride."

"Essential Health Benefits" Defined

Beginning in January 2014 all new insurance plans — whether they are offered through the private, group, or exchange markets — will be required to cover what the government believes are "essential health benefits."

This rule mandated by the ObamaCare law effectively creates a new national standard for health insurance, raising the quality of coverage for all Americans.

As discussed in the chapter on the exchanges, the list of essential health benefits has not yet been decided by the Department of Health and Human Services, but we do know that it will be similar to the list of benefits covered in the typical employer-based plan of today.

We also know that each plan must at the very least cover 60 percent of the medical costs, on average, of its enrollees (i.e., the minimum level of coverage represented by the "Bronze" plan sold through the exchanges).

While this new rule seems reasonable enough on the surface, it will, in conjunction with other ObamaCare rules, prevent insurance companies from offering bargain-basement "Mini-Med" plans to consumers, plans which have historically been profitable for them and attractive to many American consumers and businesses.

Mandating essential health benefits is a little bit like the government outlawing motorcycles because they offer less protection in an accident than an automobile. Such a requirement would undoubtedly reduce injuries and deaths on the road, but it would also encroach on the choices that Americans have always been free to make for themselves.

Many ObamaCare rules make a similar tradeoff in favor of more protection, generating opposition from those who wish to retain the range of choices that have been available to them in the past.

"Essential Benefits" Update

In November 2012 the Department of Health and Human Services announced more details about the essential benefits that all non-grandfathered insurance plans must include as of January 1, 2014.

In each of their plans, insurers must provide benefits in 10 broad categories as follows:

1. Ambulatory patient services

2. Emergency services

3. Hospitalization

4. Maternity and newborn care

5. Mental health and substance use disorder services (including behavioral health treatment)

6. Prescription drugs

7. Rehabilitative and habilitative services and devices

8. Laboratory services

9. Preventive and wellness services and chronic disease management

10. Pediatric services, including oral and vision care

While all states in the country must offer essential benefits in each of the above categories, the amount of coverage within each state will vary depending on the "typical employer plan" in the state.

For example, some states under the new ObamaCare mandate may cover treatment by chiropractors, but some may not because such coverage isn't "typical" in those states. In most cases, the largest plan by enrollment in the state's small group market will establish the state-specific benchmark required under the new law.

States will have the option, however, to use any of the three largest state or federal employee health benefit plans by enrollment or the largest insured commercial health maintenance organization (HMO) to create their essential benefits benchmark. If a state refuses to create the benchmark on its own, the default benchmark will be based on the largest plan by enrollment in the state's small group market.

In addition, if a state's essential benefits benchmark plan does not provide benefits in one or more of the 10 benefit categories, the state or the Department of Health and Human Services will supplement the benchmark plan so that they are included.

There will be some variance in the essential benefits you get with your insurance plan depending on the state you live in, but the coverage levels in each of the 10 benefit categories will probably come close to the numbers in the table below, which represent the 50-state average across the country.

TAB. A-1: **TYPICAL EMPLOYER PLAN (50-STATE AVERAGE)**		
Provided Service or Care	**3 Largest Small Group Plans**	**Federal Employee Plans**
Ambulatory Patient Services		
Primary Care Visit to Treat an Injury or Illness	100%	100%
Specialist Visit	100%	100%
Other Practitioner Office Visit (Nurse, Physician Assistant)	99%	100%
Outpatient Surgery Physician/Surgical Services	100%	100%
Outpatient Facility Fee (e.g. Ambulatory Surgery Center)	100%	100%
Home Healthcare Services	100%	90%
Skilled Nursing Facility	97%	100%
Emergency Services		
Emergency Room Services	100%	100%
Emergency Transportation/Ambulance	100%	100%
Urgent Care Centers or Facilities	100%	100%
Hospitalization		
Inpatient Hospital Services (i.e. Hospital Stay)	100%	100%
Inpatient Physician and Surgical Services	100%	100%
Maternity and Newborn Care		
Prenatal and Postnatal Care	95%	100%
Delivery and All Inpatient Services for Maternity Care	95%	100%
Mental Health and Substance Abuse		
Mental/Behavioral Health Inpatient Services	95%	100%
Mental/Behavioral Health Outpatient Services	95%	100%
Substance Abuse Disorder Inpatient Services	94%	100%
Substance Abuse Disorder Outpatient Services	95%	100%

continued on next page...

TAB. A-1: **TYPICAL EMPLOYER PLAN (continued)**		
Provided Service or Care	**3 Largest Small Group Plans**	**Federal Employee Plans**
Prescription Drugs		
Generic Drugs	84%	100%
Preferred Brand Drugs	84%	100%
Non-Preferred Brand Drugs	82%	86%
Specialty Drugs	85%	100%
Rehabilitative and Habilitative Services		
Outpatient Rehabilitation Services	100%	100%
Habilitation Services	59%	100%
Durable Medical Equipment	99%	100%
Laboratory Services		
Diagnostic Test (X-Ray and Laboratory Tests)	99%	100%
Imaging (CT and PET Scans, MRIs)	100%	100%
Preventive and Wellness		
Preventive Care/Screening/Immunization	100%	100%
Pediatric		
Dental Check-Up for Children	5%	40%
Vision Screening for Children	60%	20%
Eye Glasses for Children	8%	0%

Source: Department of Health and Human Services

The numbers in Table A-1 do not represent the level of essential benefits coverage you will have in your plan, but rather the typical levels of coverage now across the country in plans that have high enrollment.

Categories where coverage levels are deficient (e.g. pediatric care) will be supplemented in order to meet federal requirements. For example, benchmark plans that do not include pediatric vision services will need to be bolstered with benefits equal to those provided under the federal employee plan with the largest enrollment. The same goes for pediatric dental services.

While the essential benefits mandated under ObamaCare will not guarantee 100 percent coverage of all 10 healthcare categories, they represent a large expansion of benefits to millions of Americans who do not have broad coverage. Right now, for instance, 62 percent of households that buy their own health insurance do not have maternity coverage and 34 percent do not have mental health coverage. They will now, thanks to ObamaCare.

"Cadillac" Tax May Soon Be a "Chevy" Tax

The authors of ObamaCare wanted everyone to have health insurance, but not too much of it.

Such was the basis of one of its most important components — the excise tax on so-called "cadillac" health insurance plans. During the debate over the law, proponents targeted health plans that provided large benefit packages, arguing that these were held by high executives and the wealthiest who could afford to pay more.

They were worried that these extravagant plans promoted excessive healthcare consumption, which in turn drove up costs for all Americans.

To rectify this "over-utilization" of the healthcare system, ObamaCare imposes a heavy 40 percent excise tax on "Cadillac" plans that exceed a certain threshold. While this tax sounds reasonable on the surface, there is a problem. Despite what the label "Cadillac" implies, expensive health insurance plans that provide sweeping coverage are held by a broader range of people than Wall Street tycoons and wealthy industrialists.

The higher price paid for them is often a function of the holder's age, health status or insurance risk, not his or her net financial worth. Many union workers, for instance, have plans that would fall into the "Cadillac" category, and this is one reason unions opposed the tax. Firefighters, police officers, oil rig workers, and others employed in hazardous professions also require expensive insurance because their jobs are dangerous and produce a higher-than-normal risk of injury.

How will the new "Cadillac" tax work exactly? Beginning in 2018, health insurance plans that exceed $10,200 in premiums for an individual or $27,500 in premiums for a family (excluding dental and vision coverage) will be taxed at a rate of 40 percent above the threshold.

The excise tax will not be paid directly by consumers, but insurers. Critics of the tax say it will simply be passed on to employers and employees. They also point out that the tax is deceptive. Although the thresholds that trigger the tax may not seem very high today, five years from now they will seem less so since they will not be adjusted upward for inflation.

TAB. A-2: **INCREASED MEDICARE HOSPITAL INSURANCE TAX (2013 & AFTER)**			
	Plan Value	**Before ObamaCare**	**After ObamaCare**
Individuals	< $10,200	0.00%	0.00%
	> $10,200	0.00%	40%
Families	< $27,500	0.00%	0.00%
	> $27,500	0.00%	40%

*Tax imposed on amount above plan value on the insurer who issues it.

What portion of American households will be affected by the "Cadillac" tax? At first glance, the answer would seem to be not many. But much will depend on how fast healthcare premiums rise between now and 2018, when the new tax is supposed to take effect.

If you live in a state where health insurance is expensive, your risk of having to pay the "Cadillac" tax will be increased since today you are closer to the threshold than those in other states.

Soon after the law was passed in 2010, Towers Watson, a global professional services company, concluded that the new excise tax "will affect more than 60 percent of large employers' active health plans by the provision's 2018 effective date."

"The original concept of the excise tax was to penalize employers with excessively rich health benefit plans," said Randall Abbott, a senior consultant for Towers Watson. "Assuming even reasonable annual plan cost increases to project 2018 costs, many of today's average plans will easily exceed the cost ceiling primarily directed at today's 'gold-plated' plans."

Similarly, a recent study by the Pioneer Institute, a conservative think tank, estimated that more than half of the workers in Massachusetts (where health insurance costs more than any other state in the country) will have to pay the "Cadillac" tax.

By its estimate, business employees could end up paying an additional $86,905 in tax from 2018 to 2028 (about $8,000 a year), assuming the financial burden is passed on to them by their employer. A teacher who makes less might end up paying an additional $20,807 (about $2,000 a year) during the same period.

Clearly, it might be time to change the name of this controversial provision of ObamaCare to the "Chevy" tax, as it is likely to affect many middle class Americans.

Projecting the national impact of the new excise tax, the Congressional Budget Office expects that the "Cadillac" plan tax will generate $32 billion (or about 3 percent of ObamaCare's funding) during its limited two years of operation within the law's current budget, with $12 billion raised in 2018 and $19 billion raised in 2019.

Assuming ObamaCare survives into the 2020s, the tax on "Cadillac" plans is likely to become one of the new healthcare system's biggest revenue sources. Its importance should not be underestimated, especially if it impacts millions of more Americans than is currently anticipated.

Beginning in 2013 employers will be required for the first time to list the value of the health insurance they provide on workers' IRS W-2 forms that document earnings for the year. It's one small step from there to slap a new tax on healthcare benefits.

What Is A Health Insurance Exchange?

Simply put, a health insurance exchange is a marketplace very much like your neighborhood supermarket. When you need groceries, you visit your store to buy the products you need based on what's offered and the price. A health insurance exchange works the same way except the product isn't milk or cereal, but health insurance.

Each state must have an exchange and for any state that refuses to create one for its residents by 2014 (some have already threatened non-compliance) the federal government will create and manage it for them. Given the opposition from many states, fueled mostly by their dissatisfaction with the expansion of Medicaid, federally run exchanges are likely in some states.

As of mid-2012 only sixteen of the nation's 50 states had begun to create an ObamaCare health exchange. According to the non-partisan Kaiser Family Foundation, 25 states have already announced they will not create an exchange, including Alaska. Gov. Sean Parnell said that "allocating state dollars and personnel to design and implement an exchange is the most expensive option." In other words, he wants Washington to pick up the full cost for its creation and operation.

Update On Health Insurance Exchanges

In December 2012, Tennessee's Republican Gov. Bill Haslam announced that his state would not create a health insurance exchange of its own, which each state is empowered to do under the ObamaCare law. His is among the 25 states in the country that are refusing to participate in building an exchange — a startling level of non-participation in what is the central nervous system of the nation's new healthcare system.

Only 18 states and the District of Columbia have agreed to create and manage a health insurance exchange within their own borders. Another seven states are planning on partnering with the federal government to get their exchanges up and running. All ObamaCare exchanges are scheduled to open October 1, 2013, to enable consumers to buy health insurance plans that become operative on January 1, 2014.

In refusing to build its own exchange, Tennessee's governor voiced a complaint that has been expressed by other governors who have made the same decision. He blamed the White House for poor management of the process. He told the Nashville Business Journal: "The Obama administration has set an aggressive timeline to implement exchanges, while there is still a lot of uncertainty about how the process will actually work. What has concerned me more and more is that they seem to be making this up as they go."

Gov. Chris Christie of New Jersey told Jon Stewart on The Daily Show something similar, explaining why he vetoed an exchange that would have been run by his state: "I don't want to do it right now . . . Here's the issue, and why I vetoed it. I'm asking them a bunch of questions about how much this is going to cost and everything else, and they won't answer my questions . . . I'm not going to do this now . . . The law permits you always to change back to a state exchange if you want to. And what I've said to them is . . . if you can't give me all the information, you run it."

What does all of this mean for you? The most likely result is that the exchange in your state could be delayed and begin operating some time after October 1, 2013. Even if the exchange in your state opens up on time, there could be significant problems with its ability to serve customers, especially if the federal government is forced to run the exchange. While the federal government has the financial means to build the exchanges, it could have difficulty running them given the complexities of each state's specific healthcare laws.

There is another major problem looming on the horizon. Because of a mistake in how the law was written, exchanges set up by individual states are empowered to offer financial subsidies to those with lower incomes, but those set up by the federal government are not permitted, at least explicitly, to do the same thing. As of late 2012, the Internal Revenue Service appears to be ignoring this inconsistency, making it likely that federally run exchanges will offer subsidies when they begin to operate. But someone will likely file a law suit over the issue, forcing the courts to resolve the matter.

The authors of ObamaCare assumed that there would be widespread acceptance of the exchanges, and that only a few states would farm out their exchange to Washington to build and manage. That assumption has proved wrong, making the roll out of the nation's new healthcare system much more difficult than what was envisioned.

TAB. A-3: **STATE DECISIONS CONCERNING OBAMACARE HEALTH INSURANCE EXCHANGES**			
States That Have Opted in (Will Build Their Own Exchanges)			
California	Colorado	Connecticut	District of Colombia
Hawaii	Idaho	Kentucky	Maryland
Massachusetts	Minnesota	Mississippi	Nevada
New Mexico	New York	Oregon	Rhode Island
Utah	Vermont	Washington	
States That Have Opted Out (Federal Government Will Run Exchanges)			
Alabama	Alaska	Arizona	Florida
Georgia	Indiana	Kansas	Louisiana
Maine	Missouri	Montana	Nebraska
New Hampshire	New Jersey	North Dakota	Ohio
Oklahoma	Pennsylvania	South Carolina	Tennessee
Texas	Virginia	Wisconsin	Wyoming
States That Have Opted Out (Federal Government Will Run Exchanges)			
Arkansas	Delaware	Illinois	Iowa
Michigan	North Carolina	West Virginia	

For the latest news and updates on the ObamaCare law,
and what it means for your healthcare, please visit
www.SurvivingObamaCare.com

INDEX

TABLES & FIGURES INDEX

Appendix A

ABOUT THE AUTHOR

Nick J. Tate is an award-winning journalist and editor who has written extensively about health and consumer affairs issues. After a fellowship at the Harvard School of Public Health, he authored "The Sick Building Syndrome." His work has also appeared in the *The Miami Herald*, *South Florida Sun Sentinel*, *Atlanta Journal-Constitution*, *Boston Herald*, Newsmax and other publications.

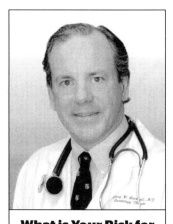

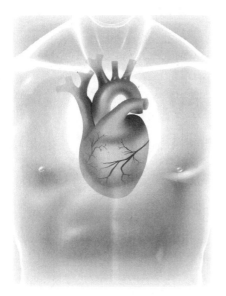

When you take the **Simple Heart Test** you'll discover:

- Your risk for developing heart disease and being a heart attack victim ...
- Which foods you can eat to protect your heart ...
- How your family's history of heart disease affects your future ...
- Whether you're getting enough exercise to strengthen your heart ...
- Your true body mass index — the percentage of your weight in relation to your height ...
- Plus much, much more!

By completing the **Simple Heart Test**, you're taking an important step in reducing your risk for becoming a victim of heart attack. Because knowing your risk for heart disease gives you a powerful starting point to take action to prevent — or even reverse — this debilitating condition.

Do not waste any more time. Complete Dr. Crandall's FREE **Simple Heart Test** now and you'll have your results in just minutes.

To take your FREE heart test, go to:
www.SimpleHeart411.com

It's easy to do! Just complete the questionnaire and you'll receive your results instantly. Plus, you'll receive Dr. Crandall's heart-healthy tips for preventing — and even reversing — heart disease.

Disclaimer: All information and results from the **Simple Heart Test** are for information purposes only. The information is not specific medical advice for any individual. The results received from taking the **Simple Heart Test** should not substitute medical advice from a health professional. If you have a heart problem or heart disease, speak to your doctor or a health professional immediately about your risk.